Because you keep asking...

Questions
about Sexuality
from
America's
College Students

Kimberly Chestnut, Ph.D.
Ranee Alison Spina, M.A.

A raz book Production
Studio City, CA 91604
Layout and design by www.urbanartdesign.com

Printed in the United States of America
First Printing: January 2014

Disclaimer: This book was written and published to help educate young adults about the complexity of sexuality. The answers to students' questions have been answered by the Authors to the best of their ability in a condensed format. Neither RAZ Productions nor the Authors shall be liable or responsible to any person or entity for any loss, damage, or injury or ailment caused, or alleged to be caused, directly or indirectly, by the information or lack of information presented in this book.

*To the courageous students
who ask questions,
when they desire to know
how to best step forward
in love, sex, dating, relationships
... and good health!*

Sexuality and

overall health

is a head-to-toe

affair.

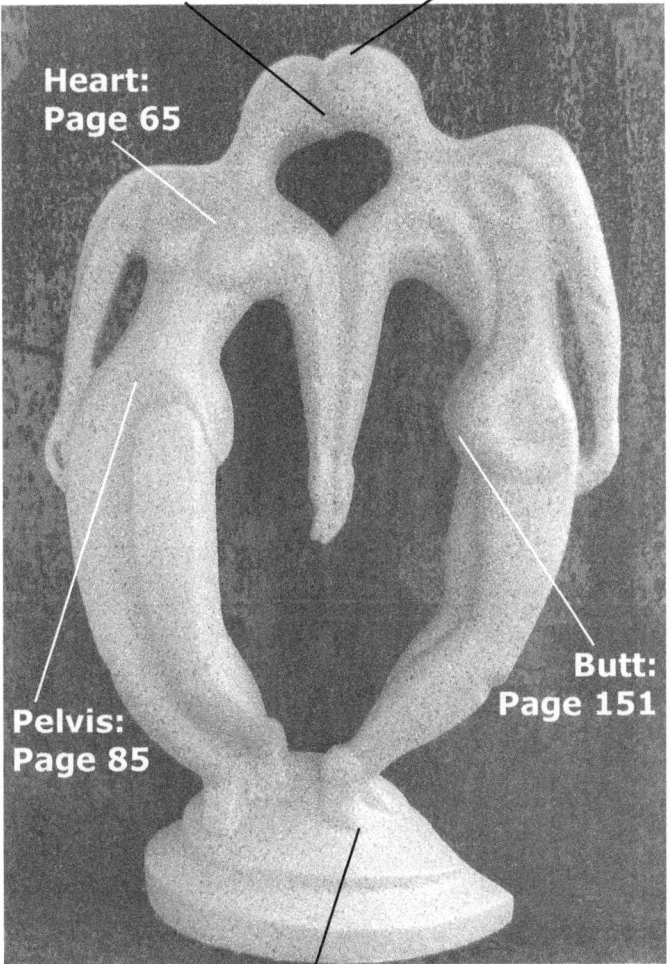

Mouth: Page 41

Head: Page 5

Heart:
Page 65

Butt:
Page 151

Pelvis:
Page 85

Toes: Page 159

SEXuality

Wow... good for you. You have questions about sexuality. We have answers. These answers represent how we have answered live Q&A with student audiences across the country.

Did you notice that we said "questions about sexuality" rather than "questions about sex?"

The reason is that sexuality encompasses a whole lot more than just having sex. It includes:

- Learning about love, desire, intimacy, and commitment
- Enhancing self-esteem
- Improving relationship skills
- Examining gender roles and stereotypes
- Recognizing and appreciating diversity
- Developing skills in life planning
- Building problem-solving skills
- Supporting healthy living habits
- Becoming a critical consumer of media messages
- Exploring spiritual aspects of sexuality
- Achieving personal success and happiness
- And, clarifying one's values...

Values play an important role when it comes to sexuality.

We hear the word "values" thrown around a lot, but what are values? Values are the messages that we have been given since birth—messages from our families, communities, friends, and the larger culture. They are complex and sometimes we don't even realize their impact until they are challenged.

Our values are the groundwork for every feeling we experience; they are an essential part of our decision making process.

We believe it's important to mention values early on, for they will likely express themselves as you read these questions and answers. You may find yourself agreeing or disagreeing with what is written—which is great—it means that you are using your critical thinking skills. That critical review is helpful in better understanding your sexuality.

As you read this book, take note of the answers that differ from how you think or feel.

Do you have any idea where your current values came from?

Some values change over time as we are exposed to new information, while other values remain the same over a lifetime.

Ultimately, we want you to have a good sense about *what* is important to you and *why* it is important to you. Are you simply following your family's or friends' beliefs?

Examine why you believe what you believe.

Make educated decisions; take in the information this book offers and change behaviors that are not aligned with good sexual health.

One more thing before you start reading the Q&A... though this book is divided into sections, we believe sexuality is "wholistic," meaning it involves the whole body. You will find some questions overlap and repetition exists due to the interconnectedness of sexuality and overall health.

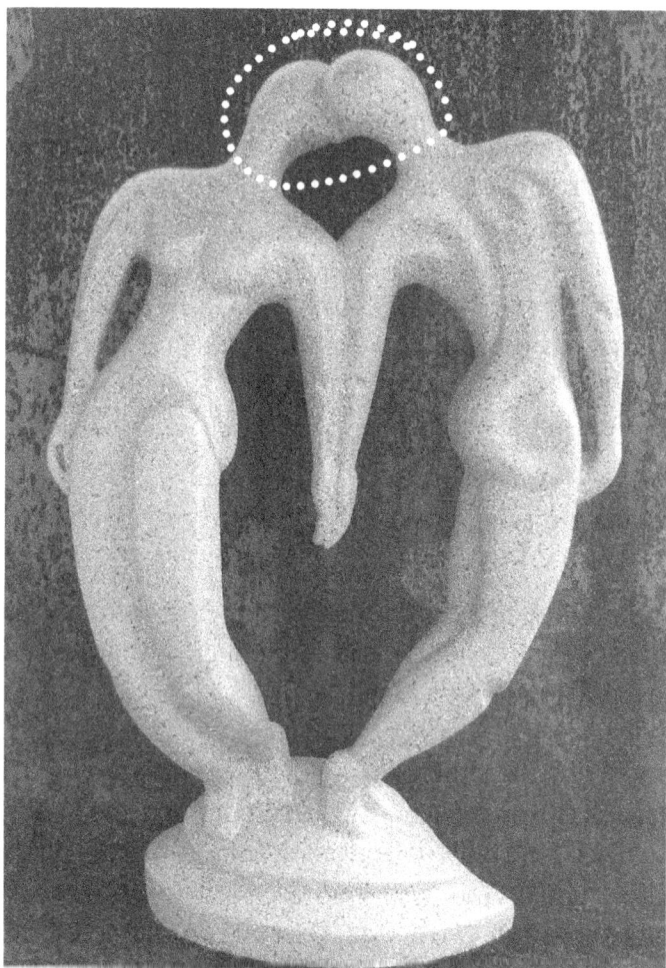

HEAD
Questions dealing with our thoughts

Did you know that Confidence is considered one of the top characteristics to describe someone who is "sexy?" Yep! Confidence is more appealing than "great legs" or "a nice butt."

If Confidence is so sexy, how come we see so little of it? *Fear of rejection? Low self-worth? A bad past experience?* No matter what the reason, it is time to rise to the occasion and understand that making healthier relationship choices leads to increased confidence.

Increased self-worth and self-respect leads to healthier sexual behavior, which leads to better overall health.

You have heard it before—respect really begins with how you feel about yourself. Do you see your strengths, as well as your weaknesses? Our ability to "see" our full selves helps us to see the complexity of others.

When a relationship first begins, it is easy to see the good in someone with whom we are infatuated, for we tend to dismiss the less appealing aspects of the person. While this is natural and somewhat "hardwired" into how we operate, we encourage you to listen to the inner voice that is telling you something about this other person. It may be positive, neutral, or negative; either way, keep listening.

If you give your time, attention, and honesty to a relationship, you deserve the same in return. If you give out a little bit of effort and commitment, you deserve back a little bit of effort and commitment from the other person.

If you are not being respected, look at how you have been treating others. *Have you been respectful?*

Also, take notice if someone does not value YOU. This person does not deserve to have you in their life. CHOOSE to spend time with people you enjoy and who make you feel good.

Q1

Can having sex make someone emotionally unstable?

Having planned, consensual sex is not likely to make someone emotionally unstable. However, the uncertainty *or assumed status* of the relationship after having sex can be stressful.

The hope is that we engage in sexual activity once we communicate about whether this is a one-time occurrence, the next step in the relationship, or an experience two people want to share without relationship expectations.

The reality is that there are emotional, physical, and for some, spiritual issues that arise when having sex. If there is uncertainty about the situation or the relationship, this can easily lead to feeling anxious, sad, guilty, or distracted. Left unchecked, these feelings could potentially lead to a sense of emotional instability.

Taking it a little further...

We as a culture must get better at
realizing the seriousness of sex,
and we must improve our education
and communication about how
and when and with whom
we want to share the experience.

Q2

How important is sex in a relationship?

Sex is another method of communication. You will discover how important sex is to you; and hopefully, you will pursue a relationship with someone who looks at sex in a similar way. Each couple perceives the importance differently.

Sexual intimacy is only one factor that impacts a couple's bonding. Notice we said "sexual intimacy" rather than "sex." Sexual intimacy includes much more than the act of sexual intercourse. It includes all behaviors where people want to achieve a physical or sexual connection such as kissing, sensual touching, discussing sexual desires, etc.

If sexual intercourse feels like too much, other options include; dry humping (outercourse), mutual masturbation, or licking/sucking. Keeping your clothes on is a good way to ensure that raging hormones don't get you caught up in the moment and lead you to something which you may regret.

**Never go against your own comfort level and give into pressure to have sexual intercourse just because your partner keeps asking, or tells you it is a condition of sustaining the relationship.*

Q3

Why is age such a big factor? Is it better for the guy to be older or for the girl to be older?

Age can be a big factor in college, because there is a significant amount of growth and development that takes place between the ages of 18 and 22. We learn so much about who we are, and up until about the mid-twenties, the human brain is still developing.

Whether the guy or the girl is older may have less to do with it than who holds the power in the relationship. Whomever is older may have an advantageous perspective over a younger partner. They have had more personal experience and may feel as though they hold the reigns in the relationship. This could be to the detriment of the younger partner, who perhaps may not yet be as aware of their own desires or as skilled in discussing the terms of the relationship.

Q4

Why do girls cheat on guys?

For the same reasons anyone cheats:

- They don't want to be in a committed relationship;

- They don't want to be monogamous;

- They made a poor choice;

- It is a pattern of behavior for them.

Ultimately, it goes back to discovering what we want in a relationship and being able to communicate with our partner. Does our partner have a similar vision? If so, there should be ongoing conversations about the health of the relationship.

Yes, communication is key, but communicating honestly is not always easy to do in daily life. Take it one moment at a time, and try your best to be honest with yourself and your significant other. We learn as we go, and no one is perfect.

Q5

After you have sex, how long should you wait to get tested for STDs?

We advise that you AND your partner get tested for STDs *before* having sex. This way, you both have a good sense about the health of the other person, *before* you rub up against them and swap bodily fluids. Yes, we do recommend barrier protection (condom/dental dam) *every* time you have sex.

An important point to make here: HIV testing has a window period—up to 6 months. It takes time for HIV to show up on a blood test. If you or your partner had sex with another person in the last 6 months, they could have been exposed to a virus that is not yet presenting in test results.

Something to think about... if you don't ask your intended partner to get tested prior to fooling around, *and use a condom/dental dam*, your head may start playing all kinds of tricks on you in regard to whether or not you caught anything. The anxiety, stress, and fear can be avoided by playing it smart.

We know that some students think it's OK to not get tested first if they plan to use condoms. Many say it is awkward to ask about STD testing; but if it's too uncomfortable to talk about safe sex, why isn't it too uncomfortable to have sex? What is really uncomfortable is when reality hits you and you ask yourself, "Did this person just give me some type of STD?"

Taking it a little further...

Do an Internet search for
comedian Patrice O'Neal's stand-up routine
about dental dams. Super funny!

Q6a

I'm a virgin and waiting for love. Is it possible?

Of course! Every option is possible. While many mainstream cultural messages portray young adults in sexual relationships, there are some which do not.

When we talk to students who are not sexually active, they seem to have a variety of friends, some who feel the same way about waiting, and others who do not.

Do exactly what makes sense to YOU and your values.

Q6b

Do you think it's OK to not listen to my fraternity brothers and wait until marriage for sex?

We have a saying...

"There is no such thing as 'have to.'"
You don't *have to* do anything.

It is *your* life, not theirs.

You have the right to structure your life any way you desire. If anyone tries to persuade you differently, or insults you in an attempt to make you feel "not normal," then ask yourself if that person can truly be called "a brother."

Surround yourself with people who support your beliefs, even if they choose a different path for themselves.

Q7

What do you do if you've been raped?

Our hope is that you know this before a rape occurs, but if you are reading this after the fact, it is never too late to address.

As soon as possible or within hours after the incident, go to the hospital and notify the police. It is extremely important that you DO NOT shower or change your clothes prior to doing either of these steps. The smallest amount of fluid or piece of hair/skin may help law enforcement prove that an assault occurred.

It is helpful to have a friend with you during this time. Receiving care and reporting rape is often a challenging process, and it may be more comforting to have emotional support. When something hurtful or scary happens to us, we tend to go into shock and have trouble thinking clearly.

If you are on a college campus, there is often free to low-cost counseling available along with other resources such as a women's center, wellness center, or victim's advocacy program through the local police department.

If you are not on a campus, there are still resources available. We advise you to get support and report the incident as soon as possible. Look into individual or group counseling sessions.

Down the road, remember to get continued emotional support any time you feel that what occurred is still causing trauma in your life.

Taking it a little further...

The Rape, Abuse & Incest
National Network (RAINN)
has a helpful website with resources,
such as:

The National Sexual Assault Hotline
1.800.656.HOPE

www.rainn.org

Q8

What exactly is date rape?

Date rape can happen on the first date, in long-term relationships, when sober or intoxicated. At this time, alcohol is the #1 date rape drug. A person can get pretty messed up by simply hanging out and drinking, or playing too many games of beer pong. As a result, decision-making skills are weakened.

Date rape is defined on RAINN.org as:

Rape is forced sexual intercourse, including vaginal, anal, or oral penetration. Penetration may be by a body part or an object. Rape can occur when the offender and the victim have a pre-existing relationship (sometimes called "date rape" or "acquaintance rape"), or even when the offender is the victim's spouse. It does not matter whether the other person is an ex-boyfriend or a complete stranger, and it does not matter if you've had sex in the past. If it is nonconsensual this time, it is rape. (Be aware that a few states still have limitations on when spousal rape is a crime.)

FACT:
You cannot give sexual consent while you are intoxicated because your judgment is impaired.

Sex and alcohol don't mix. This will be hard for some people to accept, because in the movies and in the media, we often see alcohol depicted as something that is part of a typical romantic evening.

Alcohol decreases your sexual functioning. Bodily responses are blocked. Though we may feel less inhibited, there is less turn-on, less responsiveness to being touched, and more difficulty achieving orgasm. Let us remind you that sex has no expiration date; you can always do it another day.

Here are recommendations to avoid date rape:

1. Decide earlier in the night if you want to be available to drink or available to potentially hookup, because you really shouldn't do both.

2. Do not take an open drink from someone you don't know well. Yes, it is quite easy for someone to obtain a date-rape drug, slip it into your drink, and take advantage of you.

3. Never leave your drink unattended. If you get up to dance or go to the restroom, have a friend watch your drink, or if you have to, take it with you.

If you feel like you have been sexually assaulted, get support as soon as possible. (Review Q7.)

Here are recommendations to avoid being accused of date rape:

1. Make sure you get consent from your date. Actually ask her (or him) if she (or he) wants to participate in the behavior you are intending.

2. If your date is intoxicated, don't bother asking for consent, because they can't give it; so don't do it.

3. Make sure your date gets home safely no matter what time of day or night.

*Remember, if someone is asking for your consent, communicate clearly in response. Either a yes or no. They are taking the step in asking, it is your responsibility to provide a clear and distinct response.

Taking it a little further...

The last word, according to the law:

Everyone is responsible for
what they freely and willingly do
while under the influence
of drugs knowingly taken.

If you get drunk
and choose to drive,
you're legally responsible
for the outcome.

If you get belligerent
and swing at someone,
or if you rape someone,
you are still responsible.

———

**The National Collegiate
Date and Acquaintance Rape Statistics
reports that 90% of all
acquaintance rapes involve alcohol.**

Q9

Ranee, as a former marketing director, do you feel that women and men are given a poor sense of self and a depreciative body image from the fashion and diet industries?

Absolutely! One of the reasons I retired from the advertising business was because I could no longer be a part of an industry that puts forth unreal images for society to imitate.

Magazines do not have all the answers. The articles are fluff pieces about "what is sexy" or how to be "skinny" in 30 days. First, don't ever let anyone else tell you what is or isn't "sexy." Secondly, "skinny" is not healthy. "Fit" is healthy.

Did you know that many commercials on TV are from a man's point of view? Put a woman in lingerie or in a bikini and you can sell anything. More often than not, the late-night male enhancement commercials have women with massive cleavage pitching the supplements. *Men will buy the product simply because these well-endowed women claim to desire sex with a well-endowed man?*

Really? Have we become a society that believes beauty is only size zero models in bikinis with large, fake breasts, and sex is better with an extra large penis?

Culture has a HUGE impact on what we consider beautiful or sexy. Do not allow the mass media to dictate how you should feel about your height, weight, hip size, or penis size.

Each decade brings its own sense of what is stylish, hip, cool, or sexy. If you have no confidence in what YOU consider to be stylish, hip, cool, or sexy, then you'll be floundering back and forth and most likely will never be true to yourself.

Q10

Why do I sometimes feel badly about the fact that I am having sex with my boyfriend? I love my boyfriend, but there's this thing that sex is bad.

We have a lot of cultural and religious messages that state or imply that we should feel guilty about enjoying our bodies, or being sexually active without the intention to make a baby. That being said, there are also prominent messages in our culture that support educating people about their bodies and encouraging them to think critically about who they are as sexual beings.

We teach a sex-positive approach, which means that we believe humans are sexual beings from birth to death. We need to better understand how to think about our sexuality as an essential part of our health and wellness throughout our life.

This is not the first time in history when we have seen a shift in how sexuality is seen by the larger culture. Through the centuries, there have been huge swings between sex positive and sex negative approaches, based on political or religious power holders of the time.

Pope Gregory the Great, Italian Writer Dante, and Queen Victoria had enormous impact on how society viewed sexuality. If you grew up in America, you sat through elementary, middle and high school learning about our history of war, but unfortunately not our history of love.

With all the mixed messages that have been circulating around you throughout your life, it is understandable why negative feelings may arise. Explore the root of YOUR beliefs; do not allow shame or guilt to prevail just because someone else believes a behavior is "bad."

Make healthy relationship decisions that respect both partners' needs and above all, acknowledge that sexual activity is not something to be treated carelessly.

Q11

**I'm seeing someone right now and
I was told that there should be
some chase involved. Is this true?
And what can I do to
keep her interested?**

**Do girls like a guy who is a challenge?
Or a guy who is obviously
attracted to her?**

**"You're just too nice of a guy."
What does that really mean?
How much do I have to act like a jerk
before it becomes "endearing?"**

These types of questions come up often. Here's the thing... if a girl is not excited by your interest and your attention, then we would question, "How healthy are her relationship choices?" If she is continually attracted to guys who act disinterested, blow her off, or act like a jerk in her presence, she does not have Relationship Intelligence.

Think about it—we want a relationship with someone who adores us, right? The woman who balks at attention and is obviously looking to win over the disinterested, acts-like-a-jerk guy is heading down a dead-end road.

We get that a little bit of a chase is exciting at the beginning of a new relationship. Some women use it to help them distinguish between a guy with a sincere interest and someone simply looking to hookup for a quick thrill.

A smart move would be to find a more confident girl who adores the fact that you enjoy spending time with her.

*A necessary word of advice: Do not smother her. It is important to have equal time with her, and without her. She needs time for school work, activities, friends, etc., just as YOU do.

Q12

**I'm 21 years old and I think I'm coming out of the closet.
I've experimented before, but I'm afraid to tell my fraternity brothers.
What should I do?**

We are glad to hear that you want to share this important information with your brothers. Your caution is certainly understandable, and thinking strategically about how to approach the matter is a good plan.

You have probably already considered this... it would be wise to start with those whom you know are more comfortable with various lifestyles and sexual orientations. Having a friend outside of the house that can support you through your coming out process with your brothers would be helpful. We also recommend you choose someone in the fraternity you trust—an ally—and begin sharing with him, see how it goes and take it one step at a time.

When you come out to even one person, there is no way to ensure confidentiality, so be prepared that others may find out.

There are many ways to come out: personal conversations, an email, out loud at a meeting, or less personally, by having friends tell other friends or via social media. We believe there is no right or wrong way to come out; there is only the right way for you.

Throughout this process, it's always a good idea to have someone with whom you can talk. You may want to consider having more formal support, such as a campus resource professional or counselor.

Taking it a little further...

Check out the
Lambda 10 Project online resource:

http://www.campuspride.org/lambda10

Q13

How can I avoid regretting my first time?

Most young adults get caught up in the "everyone else is doing it" or succumb to pressure from friends, a boyfriend, or a girlfriend. We understand the lure of sex and the feelings that arise when you're intensely attracted to someone; however, what society pushes on young adults is *not* going to increase your odds of no regrets.

We're going to challenge you to put aside what you see in movies, on TV, in magazines, or on the Internet. As you decide about *when* and *with whom* to have sex, think about the following:

1. Is this person someone who cares about your well-being?

2. Will this person be in your life 6 months from now?

3. Do you even care if he or she is in your life 6 months from now?

4. Do you know this person's sexual history and if he or she has been tested for STDs?

5. If intercourse did lead to pregnancy (even if condoms or other contraceptives were used), how would the two of you handle the situation? *Is this person mature enough to handle such a serious situation?*

A word about the first time you have intercourse, and we're calling it that on purpose, rather than the romantic term "making love." Making love to someone comes with maturity and experience; as with anything, we get better the more we learn and the more we practice. No one picks up a guitar for the first time and plays like a pro, so what makes people think that they will be fabulous lovers without education and the desire to learn about healthy sexuality?

Aside from the emotional reality of being sexually active, it is also helpful to consider the physical health aspect. Here are some hard facts:

1. The younger you become sexually active, and the increased exposure from a higher number of partners, results in a greater risk of cancer from a Sexually Transmitted Disease (STD).

2. Gonorrhea has been increasing among teens (especially because of those who mistakenly think they are protected from STDs if they only have oral sex).

3. A high percentage of freshmen have sex under the influence of alcohol and regret it the next morning.

4. The frontal lobe of our brains, which supports decision making, is not fully developed until our mid-twenties. Delay *The First Time* sexual experience and you will make more informed decisions when it comes to pregnancy and STD precautions.

5. 1 out of 5 teen girls contract an STI within one year of becoming sexually active.

6. You have THE REST OF YOUR LIFE to have sex. No need to rush into a potentially bad experience.

If you have already had a first time and regret it—you are not alone. Most of us make a decision from time to time where we wish for a backspace button to erase a mistake. The beauty is you now know what to avoid. If you are considering having sex again in the near future, think smart and act smart. This will decrease the odds that you will once again find yourself wishing for that backspace button.

Q14

Is touching a boob cheating when it means nothing to you?

Hmmm... We wonder why you touched a boob if it "meant nothing to you." *Simply because you could?* Was it because the woman had implants and you wanted to see what one felt like? Were you trying to turn the girl on? Maybe you had never touched one before?

Do you have a girlfriend who would consider it cheating? If your goal is to continue the relationship, we would suggest you adopt behaviors that respect her and make her happy. A successful relationship will be the balance between what makes you happy and what makes your girlfriend happy.

If she touched another guy's penis or butt, would you consider it cheating?

What if it meant nothing to her?

Q15

You talked about how KUI (Kissing Under the Influence) leads to some bad decisions—I get that. If alcohol makes a girl more willing, how does that translate to not-so-great sex?

G reat... so you have a willing girl now numbed by alcohol. Numb means less arousal, less lubrication, less pleasure, less ability to achieve orgasm, *and* the inability to give consent.

Adults both young and old are unaware of the sexual side effects that alcohol, smoking, pre-scription drugs, even over the counter allergy medications and antacids have on our sexual desire and sexual function.

For men who have difficulties achieving an erection, maintaining an erection, or reaching orgasm, they should look at what daily life habits may be inhibiting their sexual pleasure.

Taking it a little further...

The reality is:
our bodies and our brains
are less responsive when
we are under the influence.

Alcohol and sex are not a good mix.

Q16

How do fat guys get girls?

We're going to answer this question 2 ways as we're not sure if you think you're "fat" or if you wonder why "fat guys are getting the girls" which you are not. What is important here is you have brought up the subject of body image.

When we are not happy with our bodies, we can make foolish choices when it comes to sexual health. The self-talk, "I can't believe she likes me" or "I'll do anything to keep her" can lead us down the path of unsafe sex, painful sex, and/or emotional trauma.

It is great to be liked/loved for whom you are on the inside, but physical appearance does influence initial attraction. Do you think you're "fat" because you're not super skinny or are you uncomfortable to take off your shirt in front of others? Or, are you in an unhealthy state and need to put some serious effort into eating better and exercising more frequently? Being healthy will make you feel good about yourself and raise your confidence level.

Even if you don't have a magazine cover muscular physique, know this:
CONFIDENCE ATTRACTS WOMEN!!!

Look around you... people of all shapes and sizes are in relationships. Beauty truly is in the eye of beholder. There are some "not fat" guys who can not "get" girls, because they are not focused on being a considerate partner.

Q17

If you see a girl who looks like a supermodel, and you know that you may not be good enough, what should you do?

You're not good enough for what? Saying "Hello" to her? Smiling at her?

Most women find confidence attractive. Walking around with the mindset "I am less than" is not going to reflect confidence to the outside world.

Beauty is in the eye of the beholder (sometimes the *beerholder*), so do not decide for a woman what she may or may not find attractive.

Let's say this "supermodel" turns you down, what's the worst that could happen? She is one woman who walks this earth. It doesn't matter if 24 women turn you down; change up your strategy a bit and move on.

We understand that it doesn't feel good to be rejected, but don't ever let fear-of-failure stop you from approaching women. Many women are just waiting for you to say hello!

Q18

Do you think gay and lesbian people are born that way?

Here's what we know: Though we think we love with our heart, we actually love with our brain. The hypothalamus is an area of the brain that controls our basic desires such as hunger, thirst, and sex drive.

Research has discovered that the nucleus of the hypothalamus differs in size between heterosexual and homosexual men. We do believe that this could affect the sexual desire of a human being.

The hypothalamus is potentially only part of what may direct a person's sexual orientation. There are decades of research on the impacts of nature and nurture, and which has more influence on sexual orientation. It could be a combination of both—we continue to study genetics, influences, and culture to better understand the development of human beings.

Homosexuality has been around since the beginning of time. Less than 20% of our population considers themselves gay or lesbian.

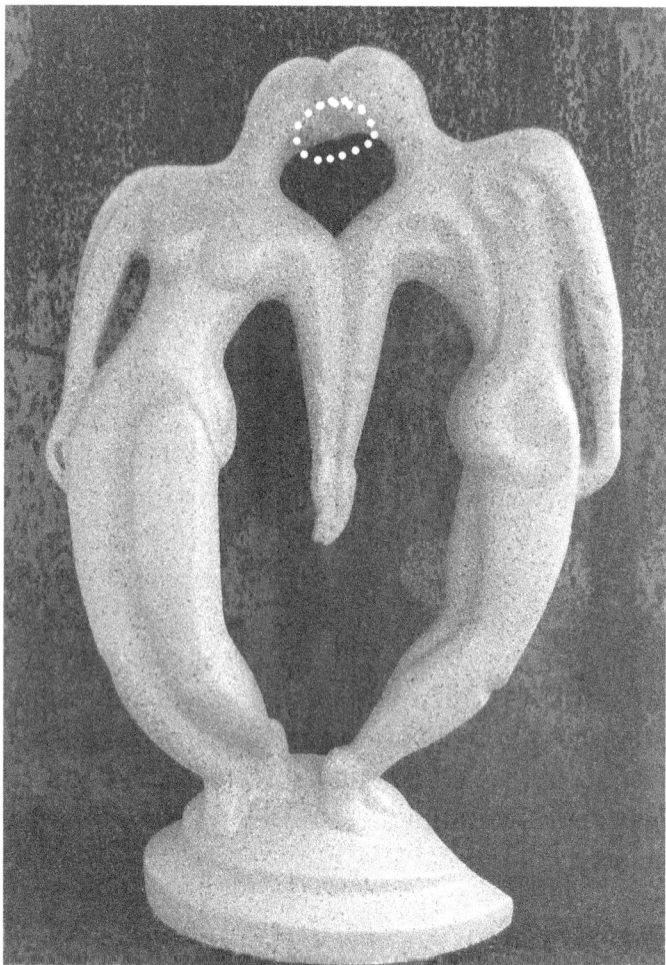

MOUTH
Questions dealing with our lips & the words that come from them

Many of you will wonder why some of the following questions have been placed in the Mouth section. The reason is because questions that deal with courage actually have more to do with your mouth than any other body part.

Courage doesn't mean not being afraid; it means feeling uneasy about a situation and communicating verbally regardless of that feeling.

It takes guts to speak up in situations that make us nervous, BUT in the end, it is worth it. Each time we speak up, it gets a little easier the next time around.

Q19

How do you deal with guy friends who always hit on you? What if you think you like them, but don't want to try dating in fear of ruining the friendship?

Hmmm... *they're your "friends" but are always hitting on you?* We're thinking the way you see the relationship isn't exactly how these guys see the relationship. Are they hanging around you because they like you more than just a friend... and, you're just not getting the hint?

Dating does not ruin a friendship; it usually is the naked bodies, swapping bodily fluids, and the love hormone oxytocin coursing through our systems that affects the relationship.

Think about what YOU want. Do you enjoy spending time with one of these guys more than the others? Be brave. Have a chat with him about taking the relationship to the next level. Given that neither of you can read minds, we suggest voicing that you want to find out if he has similar feelings.

If he says yes, great; see where it goes. If he says no, you both may feel uncomfortable for awhile, but at least you won't have to keep wondering.

Q20

What do you do when the guy confesses that he really does like you, but plays it off the next day like he never said it?

W hen exactly did he "confess" that he likes you? Was it at a party while he had a red Solo® cup in his hand?

When someone is sincere about his or her feelings for you, 24 hours isn't going to change their mind. As we said at the beginning of this section, it takes courage to share what we are thinking. If you are truly interested in this guy, ask him this:

> "Last night you told me you really like me…
> was that for real, or did you just have too
> many drinks? Because I'd like to know."

Be prepared for his response to go either way. You're taking a chance just as he did the night before.

Q21

I really like a guy, but I'm too shy to approach him about my feelings. How can I let him know how I feel without being embarrassed?

There are 3 ways we see this playing out:

1. You do nothing, which later you may regret.

2. You ask a friend to get a sense if he is interested.

3. Try something different. Find that little piece of you that can be brave for just 2 minutes to tell him you're into him. Will it be easy? No, but you can do it. You're also giving him the chance to tell you how he feels.

Fear of embarrassment and fear of rejection affect us all. Sometimes we just have to suck it up, get past our shyness or fear and take action. Our anxiety about a situation is usually much worse than reality.

Q22

I have the problem where I go out with guys (good looking ones); they keep in touch, but I never know where it's going. How do I ask them?

When guys want to see you, they'll see you. When guys want you to be their girlfriend and not see other guys, they will ask. If there has been no conversation regarding the relationship status, then bring it up.

Isn't it better to know whether or not you're on the same page rather than wonder what is going on?

*It is very important to know the status of your relationship if you are sexually active. YOU are responsible for YOUR health, so do not get conversation shy when you need to know with whom a guy is also partnering with in a sexually intimate way.

Q23

I hate the pressure I feel when a guy thinks I have to kiss him, like it's almost always expected. What can I do to get out of it, but not turn him off?

There is no such thing as "have to." You are in control of your body. If anyone attempts to make you feel differently, tell them, "That makes me feel uncomfortable. I really like you, but I'm not comfortable kissing you right now."

Hugs are an excellent way to end an evening or a date. A hug can show feelings for someone while not necessarily being of a sexual nature.

Q24

What do I do when my roommate kicks me out at 1 am to hookup with someone?

Not cool on your roomie's part. It is a good idea to have a conversation about such situations before they happen.

For example, roommates can agree to provide 24 hours notice if one would like to have the room to him or herself. This also helps to avoid regrettable choices often influenced by alcohol.

Q25

How do you tell a girl that you care for her?

Keep it simple. Consider something along the lines of:

> "I don't want to scare you off, but I wanted you to know that I think you're an amazing person and _____.
> (Fill in the blank with whatever your intentions are: to be friends, to go on a date, etc.)

You can do it! If she is meant to be a part of your life, she'll be receptive to your interest.

Q26

What do I say if the truth isn't so nice about my boyfriend's kissing style?

In order for someone to be considered a good kisser, he or she usually has a kissing style that matches our own. Obviously, your kissing partner has a very different kissing style than yours.

Kissing is a lost art and our love lives would improve greatly if we all learn to appreciate the greater intimacy that kissing encourages.

Start by asking him to slow down and concentrate only on the kiss. Tell him to allow you to kiss him in the fashion that you want to be kissed. Then, have him do to you what you just did to him. Give him time to adopt the new kissing style... *practice!* You may also want to ask him what kind of kissing technique he finds desirable.

Taking it a little further...

Did you know there are books
that give you detailed info
on how to be a fabulous kisser?
(hint, hint)

Q27

How do you tell someone you really like that some of his sexual moves aren't that good?

This happens quite a bit, for we each have a preferred sexual style. This is where good communication with your partner comes into play. Always start with the positive, "I like it when you run your fingers through my hair; do that more and stick your tongue in my ear less."

Or, you could ask him what he likes the most *and the least* about your moves and hopefully he will ask for your feedback too. If not, we encourage you to offer anyway.

Q28

How could I enhance pleasure by using my mouth? (blowjobs, rim jobs, etc.)

Sexual pleasure is about a shared experience that should include conversation about what feels good to the other person. If you only think about what you are doing to the other person, then it becomes more of a script or pattern you follow, rather than taking an interest in what your partner needs and/or wants.

Some people enjoy oral sex, others do not. Some people get turned on with anal play; others find it a turn off. Some people have never had a generous, loving partner, so they don't know what might feel good versus what does nothing to excite their senses.

Have a chat about what each other likes and focus your skills from there. Remember that safer sex calls for using a condom or dental dam when placing your mouth on anyone's genitals or anus.

Optimally, we should strive throughout our entire life to grow as a sexual human being. With each decade, comes different excitement and new learning experiences.

Q29

How do you talk to
your parents about sex?

Even parents can find sex talk awkward. They may be a little unsettled at first, but give them a chance; they will likely get in sync after a moment of consideration. Anticipating their potential initial surprise or discomfort allows you to let them have their reaction, and then you can start talking.

What type of questions do you have? *Birth control, intercourse, sexual orientation?* Are you looking for their guidance, wisdom, or help with a situation? Let them know how they can help you. No matter what is on your mind, be open to listening to what they have to say. The respect needs to be mutual, and hopefully, helpful conversation will result.

If you still need more information after the chat, check in with campus resources or a counselor. Expect complete confidentiality. Many students fail to take advantage of the great resources in their counseling center.

You won't be the first or last to ask a question pertaining to sexuality; 1 out of every 4 students is there with a question similar to yours!

Q30

I think my roommate is gay or possibly trans; what should I do?

Be kind, considerate, and communicative—just as you should be with any roommate. If you feel you want to talk specifically about sexual orientation or identity, we encourage you to be honest. Be sure to let him or her know you are unfamiliar—and maybe a little uncomfortable—with the difference in lifestyles.

One of the beauties of college is learning new things and growing personally. Discuss how you can be considerate towards one another. No doubt, there will likely be things about you that your roommate finds unfamiliar and uncomfortable.

Taking it a little further...

For information on understanding
Sexual Orientation and Gender Identity:

www.apa.org/topics/sexuality

Q31

My sorority sisters insist that oral sex isn't considered having sex with someone. Do you agree?

Nope. It's called "oral sex," not "oral exercise" or "oral studying." Hmmm... we're thinking that's because it is sexual activity (though people do need to study oral sex techniques). The term "sex" is not limited to the act of vaginal penetration.

We hear some college students say, "Blow jobs are like 2nd date activity." **Not safe and not smart.**

The 2nd time you go out with someone, or hang out with someone, we doubt you have asked about STI/STD testing. And if someone does tells you they are symptom free, it does not mean they are not a carrier. Though not as sexually exciting, condoms and dental dams do help prevent bodily fluids from mixing when giving and receiving oral sex.

Remember: You cannot see the bacteria on the back of someone's throat. What you may perceive as "harmless, safe oral sex" may give you gonorrhea—an STI that is known to easily be passed from one to another via oral sex. The bacteria is far from harmless; as of 2013, gonorrhea has progressively developed resistance to the antibiotic drugs pre-scribed for treatment.

Mouth and throat cancer can also be a result of HPV (Human Papilloma Virus) transmitted orally. HPV is usually thought to only be associated with cervical cancer, but it actually has also been transmitted orally and anally.

Wait for STI/STD test results BEFORE getting near anyone's genitals and before letting anyone get near yours.

Ladies, a word to the wise... reciprocity wins here. If you enjoy receiving oral sex, you might want to do only that which has been done to you first. ;)

Taking it a little further...

Gonorrhea cases have been increasing due to the myth that you can't get an STI when only having oral sex.

We will see more oral cancers develop due to the transmission of HPV and Gonorrhea.

Q32

Why do so many guys assume that when they try to start having sex and a girl says "I don't think so," or she is drunk, it means to keep trying?

These guys are attempting to wear the girl down with persistent pressure, especially if the girl has had some alcoholic beverages, lowering her resistance.

The bottom line is that Sexual Consent requires both of the following:

1. The pursuer needs to clearly ask, "Do you want to have sex?"

2. The respondent needs to answer crystal clear, either "YES" or "NO," not a cutesy "Maybe..." or "I don't know."

*If someone is intoxicated, they are not legally able to give consent. In other words, don't ask someone who is intoxicated to have sex with you unless you have a desire to wear an orange jumpsuit and be Bubba's girlfriend in jail.

Someone who is pushing you to have sex most likely is not concerned about your well-being.

Remember, it is YOUR BODY and you have control over it. On party nights, buddy-up and be sure to stay with friends who have your back. As we said earlier, it is a good plan to decide if the night will be about hooking up or drinking, because the two just don't mix.

There are plenty of nights when neither drinking nor hooking up has to be an option!

Q33

I have had herpes for about 2 years. Where can I get treated, and how do I tell girls who I plan to have sex with in the future?

It is important to seek out medical help as soon as possible. Through campus health services, or at a local health center, you can get connected with a doctor to review treatment options.

Some patients decide on antiviral therapy. Antiviral medication can be administered either as suppressive therapy to reduce the frequency of outbreaks or can be taken once a sore is noticed to shorten the duration of lesions. Topical medications that can be purchased over-the-counter can help minimize the duration of an oral herpes outbreak.

The frequency of recurrent genital herpes outbreaks diminishes over time in many patients. With herpes there is no cure, but good health is essential.

It is helpful to understand the triggers that can cause outbreaks and how to best handle the symptoms. Minimize outbreaks by getting adequate sleep, reducinging stress, and taking good care of your general health.

When it comes to telling girls in the future, we encourage you—as we do with everyone—to not initiate sexual activity until you have open communication about being sexually active. When you start these conversations, you can then mention that you have herpes and you are careful about managing outbreaks. You want your girl-friend to know early to help keep her healthy; share with her how you take care of yourself and what you can do together to reduce transmission.

Taking it a little further...

Planned Parenthood
has wonderful resources
for in-person visits and online.

If you visit
the Favorite Links Page on
SmartSexRocks.com,
there are helpful Internet resources listed.

Q34

What do I do if my boyfriend won't tell me how many people he has slept with?

R un? (Just kidding.) He's most likely having a hard time answering this because he has no idea what you will consider "too many." His number could be 3 or 40, but if you are looking for him to say 1 or 2, then he loses his chances of having sex with you or it changes the way you see him.

Listen to your gut, especially if something is telling you that this guy may put your emotional or physical health in danger. It might be the best time to consider finding a boyfriend who is willing to share information with you. We understand that it may be difficult and heartbreaking to move on from this guy, but the goal is to be in a relationship in which you both care and communicate about sexual health.

Taking it a little further...

Be smart.
Make sure you ask about sexual history,
safe sex practices, and testing frequency.

Do the words on the next page look and sound familiar? Probably. We hear them all the time on TV, in the movies, in the media, on the Internet, and in casual conversation. Take a good look at the words.

Are they offensive?
> *Are they negative or positive?*

The casual use of certain words can cause us to overlook their meaning. Notice that the common terms used for males can be positive, while female names are negative. Notice that the terms for sexual activity can be violent and forceful.

What ends up happening is that women are seen and treated differently than men. They are treated in a negative way.

Choose your words carefully.

MALE	FEMALE	SEXUAL ACT
Gigolo	Slut	Banged/Pounded
Casanova	Whore	Schmanged
Don Juan	Ho	Hit it & quit it
Player/Playa	Skank	F*cked
Pimp	B*tch	Get on, get off, get out
Daddy	Momma	Smash
Dude	Cum Dumster	Get it
Man	Chick	Squash
Bro	Hoochie	Screw
Fella	Hooker	Drill it
Stud	Hottie	Gettin' in it
Womanizer	Skeezer	Hooking up
Cheater	C*nt	Doin' the nasty
Manwhore	Tramp	Humping
Baller	Sketch	Turning tricks
Mack	Ratchet	Knockin' boots
A-hole	Pussies	Bumpin' uglies
Hustler	Gash	Gettin' freaky
Cock	Prostitute	Sex you up

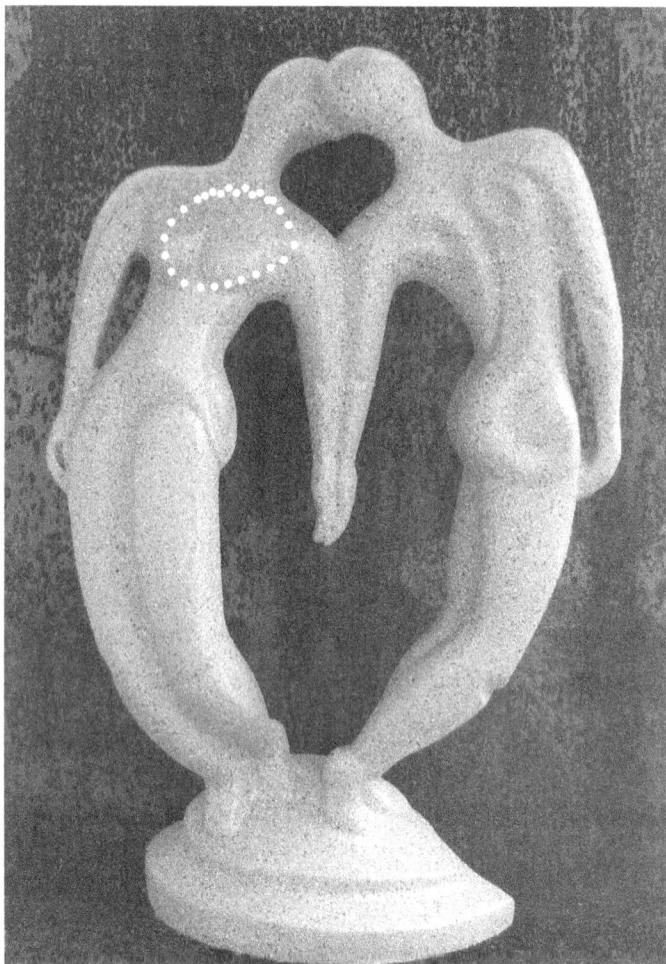

HEART
Questions dealing with love & relationships

Everything you do in life will be dependent on one thing: self-worth. Your self-worth will influence your personal relationship choices and behaviors.

Who you allow to be part of your life and how much energy you put into *someone else's success* versus *your own success* will be largely impacted by what you think you're worth.

We cannot build your self-worth, but we can share with you this fact: Relationships, with toxic people who do not have your well-being in mind, will beat you up on the inside and decrease your self-worth.

Choosing to be in a healthy relationship, where you feel your time and energy are worth it, will boost your sense of well-being and increase your self-worth.

Q35

The girl I love and have been with for 20 months lives an hour from me. It is a continual fight between us as to when I should visit. What can I do in this situation?

It isn't easy, but you have to decide on how to spend your limited time. Most of us would agree that spending a lot of time fighting is a waste of time. If you two could agree to see each other every other weekend, then you also have to agree to not make it the topic of conversation on the other weekends.

Those students who choose to leave campus every weekend are denying themselves the full experience of going away to college. We understand that you care about your girlfriend, but she still has moments to experience at her school and you have moments to experience at your school. This is it; you don't ever get to be this age at this place ever again.

This also applies to those who are in a relationship with someone who is not in college. Maybe your guy or girl works and has more free time to hang out rather than worry about coursework. Either way, your time is your own; you need to communicate your expectations and needs.

Q36

You say to kiss many girls, but how do you do it without feeling guilty or offending her? Girls won't understand!

The reason we say to "kiss many girls" is to dismiss the assumption that one kiss means an instant relationship. Just because you hang out with someone, ask her out and/or happen to kiss her, doesn't mean that the two of you are a couple. You are simply seeing if you enjoy someone's company... and the way she kisses.

If you are not interested in a serious relationship, do not lead a girl on as if you are *and* be sure to remind her if she starts acting as if she is your girl-friend. You don't have to be mean about it, just remind her that she is not your girlfriend. Allow her the opportunity to go find a guy who is looking for a committed relationship.

Q37

How do I tell a friend how I really feel about her? If she does want to take it beyond friendship, how do I deal with the person I'm in a LDR (Long Distance Relationship) with now?

How do you deal with the desire for companionship & physical closeness without seeing other people?

LDRs are GU! (Geographically Undesirable) Why? Because you're not able to have the day-to-day contact and enjoyment with that person.

Texting "<3" day after day isn't as much fun as laughing with someone in person. Obviously, you've already figured this out and now have feelings for someone who does live nearby.

Your LDR deserves a conversation about how the two of you need to date others. Be sure to end one relationship before asking someone else out. Your good friend may begin to see you differently if you are available.

Q38

**I am in a long-term relationship
with my very best friend and have
a hard time making guy friends.
It's awkward because I don't
know what kind of hanging out
is crossing the line.**

**Should he be mad if I want to go
to a club and dance with other guys?
Any suggestions or input?**

Attending football games, having lunch, going for a bike ride, hanging out with a group of friends... these are things that "friends" do that don't cross the line. Think about what you would be comfortable with him doing with a girl who is *only* his friend. What kind of dancing would you want him to be doing with "just a friend?" Would you want another girl pushing her butt back into your boyfriend's crotch? Grinding may be one of the dance moves you two decide is off limits.

Share your thoughts with him, and hopefully you come to an agreement on how to respect your relationship while maintaining other friendships. It is a good idea to have your boyfriend meet your friends; that way he knows who you are talking about when you spend time with them.

Q39

Why do guys say they want to "take a break" from the relationship, and a short time later, want to get back together again?

Guys sense 1 of 2 things:

1. They are aware something is just not right with the relationship and want out without having to confront you with the break-up conversation, or...

2. They are looking to be available for another girl, and therefore, won't be technically cheating on you.

When these guys get lonely, they say they want to get together again. Most likely, the process will repeat unless you decide that being the default go-to-girl isn't good enough for you. The next time a guy wants to get back together after "taking a break," simply say, "not interested!"

Q40

How do you research the kind of woman you should choose?

This is actually a great question. Many times, people simply stay with the first person for whom they have feelings, even though that person is not a complementary match. "Complementary" means that which goes well with you—your likes, dislikes, values, beliefs, etc.

The *only* way to figure out who goes well with you is to spend time with different people and compare how you feel. You will notice who makes you feel good and who brings you down. No one fits us perfectly as most fairytales lead us to believe.

Don't wait for "perfect" and be prepared to have some good and not-so-good finds along the way. It is part of the process; you'll figure out what's good for you by eliminating that which does more harm than good.

And don't be fooled into thinking the grass is greener on the other side; all grass needs to be watered and cared for, so be prepared to invest time and energy into a relationship no matter who you choose.

Q41

What should I do
if I like a girl and she likes me,
but she can't decide between me
and another guy she also likes?

You and this girl are dating. She is also dating the other guy.

"Dating" means that you are going out socially with someone with whom you have a romantic interest. It doesn't mean kissing, having sex with, hooking up with, or that you are in a committed relationship.

There is no commitment until one of you decides to ask for a monogamous relationship. Maybe you should take her lead and date some other girls? Or you could ask for her exclusive commitment. If she isn't saying yes, she is saying no.

If you are sexually active, the monogamy talk is very important to your health. Multiple, concurrent, sexual partners increases your chance of contracting an STD/STI.

Q42

Is there still hope for a handsome college guy who has never been kissed by a girl? Will someone want to date me?

Today's TV shows, movies, and magazines put forth the perception that "everyone" is hooking up or has a significant other. SO NOT TRUE!

You're in college to get an education, not to worry about being in a relationship.

There is no doubt you will find what you are looking for—we just have to wait a little longer than we expect. If you're lucky, you will have many relationships! Yes, *lucky!* Because each relationship teaches us something about ourselves.

Q43

Why do young guys like older women?

Here are 3 reasons for this attraction:

1. The belief that older women can teach a younger guy something that will make him a better lover.

2. They are looking to check off one of their boxes:
   - ☑ Over 35
   - ☑ Blonde
   - ☑ Brunette
   - ☑ Redhead
   - ☑ _____ (fill in the blank)

3. There was an event in their childhood development that triggers the sexual attraction (for example, being attracted to a friend's Mom.)

Remember, not all young guys like older women.

Q44

Are threesomes really that good?

Threesomes are a sexual experience some people choose to explore. It is one of many ways to explore sexuality. Be aware that sexual experience between two people can be tricky; it can be even more difficult with three.

If it feels uncertain or you don't really want to—*and would only do it to make someone else happy*—then don't. Honor yourself and YOUR values above those of others.

Q45

I have the perfect boyfriend, but how do you know if you are ready to really be in love?

And how do you tell him that you love him more than anything, but need a little space and time to be 20 without giving up something great?

We can't help with whom we fall in love, but we can direct what we do with those feelings. Being in love is exhilarating—especially the dizzying, exciting effects of first love.

Here's the hard truth:
The area of our brain used for decision making isn't fully formed until our mid-twenties.

With this in mind, how could—*or why would*—anyone want to make a decision too early about who they are going to love for the rest of their life?

That space and time you talk about needing? We agree with it! Take all of your 20's to discover who you are, what makes you happy, and who would make a "perfect man" for you.

Make a commitment to yourself before making a commitment to someone else.

Q46

If you're truly in love with someone, what's wrong with living together and sharing your life, especially in your 20's?

It depends on what you want the end result to be—marriage or just someone to live with during your 20's. *Do you both have the same expectations?*

You are not immune to the statistics of cohabitation. Couples who live together prior to marriage are less likely to survive to their 10 year anniversary.

If you are like most 20-somethings, what you want at age 21 will drastically change by age 29. Set yourself up for success in love and life. Use your 20's to discover you—what you like and dislike—before you make a commitment to anyone for the rest of your life. Someone you "truly love" deserves a well-informed decision of commitment.

Q47

How would you define dating in college and when does it go from just seeing each other to a relationship?

When people are sexually active, many refer to it as "seeing someone," "hooking up" or "in a committed relationship."

What most of you are missing is that dating actually has a purpose. Dating is not asking someone over to your dorm room to watch a movie and hopefully have sex. Dating is not seeing someone at a party and over a red Solo®cup asking them to come home with you. Dating is asking someone to spend time with you in order to get to know him or her better. Having a cup of coffee together, going on a hike, going to a basketball game, etc.—these are ways we can interact to see if we enjoy being with this person.

We hear girls say, "I slept with that guy and he is such a jerk." Most likely, they would have found out he was a jerk if they had spent time with him prior to sleeping with him. We understand he is really sexy, but jerks can be sexy too.

Any sexual activity brings about emotional and physical risk; imagine if something happens like getting pregnant even with condom use. If you took that risk with a sexy jerk, well, don't be surprised when he acts like a jerk and doesn't own up to his responsibility.

An intimate relationship occurs when 2 people sit down and communicate out loud that they each would like to be in a relationship and no longer date or hookup with other people. Without this verbal confirmation, you have no idea if someone is interested in a committed, monogamous relationship.

Don't assume just because someone is willing to have sex with you, he or she is not seeing anyone else.

Q48

What are questions you should bring up or discuss with your partner before you get married (or decide to get married/engaged)?

There are many topics to discuss in order to increase your chances of happily ever after. Here is a partial list to get you started.

1. What does marriage mean to you?

2. How will the finances be handled?
   - How much can you spend individually, as a couple, and how much money will be saved, if any?
   - Does someone make significantly more money than the other? If so, how will that affect the questions above?

3. Where do you want to live and in what type of housing?

4. Who will be responsible for cooking, cleaning, laundry, yard work, etc?

5. Will we have pets?

6. Do we spend time with each other's families? How much and how often?

7. Will we both keep friendships with people of the opposite gender?

8. Do you want to start a family? If so, when?
   - How many children do you want?
   - Where do you want to raise this family?
   - Will one parent stay home with the children?
   - How do you believe a child should be disciplined?
   - Will there be spiritual teachings for the children?
   - Will a male child be circumcised?
   - What happens if we are unable to conceive children? Do you believe in adoption?

9. If an unintended pregnancy occurrs, what will we do?

10. Who will initiate sex? Are we free to say no to sex?

11. How often will we engage in sexual behaviors with each other?

12. What will be included/excluded in the boundaries of our sexual activities?
    Anal sex, oral sex, masturbation (self or mutual), pornography, sex on the Internet, bondage, S&M, sex toys, sex clubs, fetishes...

Because you keep asking...

$$sex \neq love$$

sex ≠ a relationship

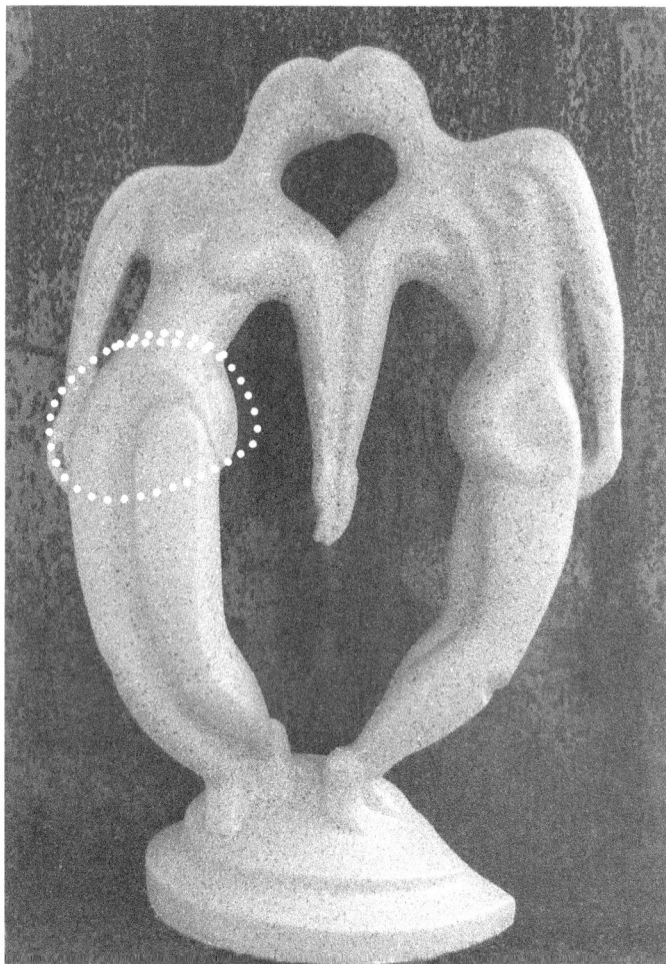

PELVIS
Questions dealing with genitals, orgasm, STDs pregnancy & condoms

You will find that this is the largest section of the book. That's probably not a big surprise given our culture's focus on anatomy when it comes to talking about sexuality. As you have read by now, sexuality is about much more than what is between the legs! Still, what is between the legs—and how it affects the rest of our body—is very important. This section will take us through orgasm, sexually transmitted infections, pregnancy, and much more.

Because you keep asking...

orgasm

Q49

Why is it so much harder for girls to have an orgasm than guys?

A man's penis is fully exposed on the exterior of his body. It is a surface area of [on average] 5-7 inches in length and 4-6 inches in circumference when erect. This total surface area has nerve endings available to experience sexual pleasure; the ease of access to the area allows for more easily-achievable orgasms.

The female body also has surface area with nerve endings that can be stimulated; it just isn't protruding out of the body with the same ease of access.

Most people don't know that the clitoris actually has legs—yes, legs—which run below the surface tissue just above and around the sides of the vulva. An analogy that may help is to think of the clitoris as a wish bone, with the visible part of the clitoris being at the top and the legs running down the sides. You can stimulate the clitoris by providing pressure through clothing in this area. Many think you have to touch the clitoris and clitoral hood, but you don't; women can experience orgasms through outercourse.

Q50

Is it possible for a girl to be unable to have an orgasm? How do you know if you are having one?

You are not alone in your struggle to understand orgasm. In fact, many older women have shared that they have never had an orgasm.

Many of us don't know how our body works to achieve an orgasm. Did you know that the brain and spinal column play a big part in orgasms? The spinal column transmits sensations between your brain and your genitals.

Let's start with the clitoris, because more women achieve orgasm via contact to this genital area versus repetitive vaginal penetration. If a woman has an intact clitoris (meaning it has not been significantly injured or circumcised/female genital mutilation) then she should be able to achieve orgasm with adequate stimulation.

However, the ability to achieve orgasm does not depend solely on your physical condition; having an orgasm can be heavily influenced by how someone is feeling or what they are thinking about while engaging in sexual activity. This is one reason that women often find it challenging to achieve orgasm.

Women may not be emotionally or mentally available and this can make it more challenging to be focused on how the body is feeling and if the pleasure will result in orgasm.

For example, if you are stressed out about exposing your naked body, you may not be open to the experience of how it feels to be lovingly touched.

There are many stressors that can inhibit sexual pleasure and satisfaction. For optimal sexual health, these stressors must be acknowledged and addressed:

- pain
- fatigue
- anxiety
- fear
- depression
- medication
- negative past experiences
- recreational drugs
- power/control issues
- loss of interest in partner
- hormonal influences
- low self-image

Given orgasms vary in intensity, location, and scenario, it is impossible and inadequate to give one example of what it would be like for everyone or every time. We define orgasm as a pleasurable bodily experience of muscle tension and release that supports overall well-being.

The stimulation should feel good and you should be able to feel it building in intensity. Heart rate increases, breathing becomes more rapid, blood flow to the vulva increases, breasts swell, and the body heats up inside and out. At the height of the intensity, the body will release the built up tension. The release feels like a sudden explosion, but upon examination, it's really a series of waves. Ejaculation in men and women happens when those muscle "waves" pulse through the body and push fluid through whatever tube or tissue it happens to be in which leads to an exit.

Know that you and your partner are both entitled to experience pleasure and possibly orgasm. Don't feel like once one is done, the party is over. What you want each time you sexually connect with someone will vary, but be aware if your partner has had their desires met too.

There are some selfish and clueless lovers out there; so choose partners who understand that it is a shared experience.

If you feel like you have not had an orgasm yet, you are not alone. We encourage you not to worry; you will continue to learn about your body. Focus on enjoying all that you do experience and know that there is much pleasure in various forms of sexual interaction (orgasm is far from being the only good part).

Sexual activity, experienced alone or with someone else, is complex. This is such a common question that there are many books addressing the issue.

Taking it a little further...

For further reading on female orgasm
and pleasure, look into the works of
Sheri Winston, who is a unique sex educator
with great information.

Q51

Why is it that when I masturbate I can reach orgasm, but during sex I can't?

There are a few common reasons why this might be the case. If you have female genitalia, a vagina and clitoris, it is often easier to achieve orgasm via masturbation, because attention can be focused on the clitoris or a combination of the clitoris/vagina where more women achieve orgasm.

More often than not, a partner simply moving his penis in and out will not provide optimal stimulation for a woman to experience orgasm.

Another common situation for limited orgasm with a partner can pertain to the emotional realities of being sexually active. Possible thoughts associated with STIs/STDs, unintended pregnancy, body image, etc. can all influence how "available" we are to experience pleasure to the point of orgasm when with another (as we mentioned in response to Q50).

If you have a penis and cannot reach orgasm during sex with a partner, your mind may be too consumed with other thoughts. We ask you to consider if you are overwhelmed with school or work, or perhaps you're watching too much pornography during self-stimulation. Some men who excessively watch pornography, can only become aroused by the less-than-life-like images many flicks contain.

Sexual health includes the ability to be intimate with a real-life partner. (Though great for masturbation, Fleshlights, Wrap-Around Sallies, blow-up dolls, and porn star vulva/anus replicas do not count as partners.)

Sexually Transmitted Diseases
&
Sexually Transmitted Infections

Will you be one of the millions to catch an STI/STD this year?

Teenage girls in the 15-19 age group
have higher Chlamydia and Gonorrhea
rates than any other age group
and teen boys.

Almost half of all new
sexually transmitted diseases
are in teens and young adults
ages 15 to 24 years old.

Q52

Is there a big difference between STDs and STIs?

In the past 10-15 years, the use of the term sexually transmitted infections (STIs) versus sexually transmitted diseases (STDs) has been used for a couple reasons.

1. Infections can be symptom-free, yet still active and contagious. Additionally, bacterial infections (for example, chlamydia, syphilis, gonorrhea) or parasites (for example, trichomoniasis, lice, crabs) are sexually transmitted and can be cured with treatment.

2. Viruses (for example, HPV, HIV, herpes, hepatitis) that are transmitted can be treated but not cured, therefore qualifying as a disease.

The term STI is used more frequently due to the fact that all STDs start out as an STI, but not all STIs turn into an STD.

Note: Due to the overuse of antibiotics, Gonorrhea is one of the bacterial infections that is progressively becoming antibiotic-resistant.

Q53

Does shaving pubes get rid of crabs?

No, you have to get a topical prescription to treat crabs. Please see a doctor as soon as possible to get a full treatment plan.

Do not have ANY sexual contact until the doctor has confirmed that you no longer have crabs.

Q54

Are there STI/STD testing places on campus, besides testing for H.I.V?

Many colleges and universities have a student health center where STI/STD screening is available. If you are not in school, or your school does not offer this service, look online for what options you have locally. Another option can be to ask your primary doctor for a full screening.

Once sexually active, it is very important to have an annual health screening. If your doctor does not offer to test for STIs/STDs, ask to have it done.

Women, when visiting a gynecologist, be sure to ask about testing for various STIs/STDs. Pap-smears are not always done, but if you have a specific question or concern, please ask your doctor; it is their job to help you.

Please note: pap-smears test for abnormal cell development such as HPV and cervical cancer. A pap-smear does not test for any other sexually transmitted infections or diseases.

Many schools or health clinics can treat you without informing your parents. Parental insurance does not need to be used if your screening is covered by the school or if services are offered at a low cost that you can pay on your own.

Q55

So I hear there are multiple forms of herpes. Which is which? And can you cross contaminate?

There are two forms of herpes that are transmitted sexually: Herpes simplex virus 1 and 2. Herpes simplex virus 1 originates orally, and herpes simplex virus 2 orginates genitally. However, they can be transferred to other areas of the body.

If someone with oral herpes performs oral sex there is the chance that the receiving person could contract herpes genitally. And vice versa, if you perform oral sex on someone who has genital herpes, you could end up getting herpes orally. For this reason, it is always recommended to use condoms when performing oral sex on a penis and use a dental damn when performing oral sex on a vulva. Essentially, while there are two forms, the distinction is minimal, because they both can be contracted in both areas.

Q56

Is actual intercourse the only way to get an STD?

Nope.

Sexually transmitted infections and diseases can be transferred various ways. Many are transferred via male ejaculate, vaginal secretions, and blood. Others can be transmitted via skin-to-skin contact. HIV can be transmitted to babies via breast milk from an HIV positive mother.

Avoid becoming one of the millions of students each year who transmits or becomes infected with a sexually transmitted infection. Information on transmission, prevention, symptoms, and treatment is widely available on the Internet or a course textbook on human sexuality.

Taking it a little further...

5 myths about STDs
www.TeensHealth.org

Sexually Transmitted Diseases
www.cdc.gov/std

Q57

Is a yeast infection contagious?
I think my boyfriend gave me one.

Yes. Yeast infections can be sexually transmitted. Your boyfriend can pass the infection to you, and you can pass the infection to him. Similar to STIs, yeast infections can go back and forth between partners if sexual activity is not halted while both partners are treated.

If you did not have a yeast infection, you may want to ask your boyfriend if he has been on an antibiotic or is sexually active with other people.

Antibiotics make us more susceptible to yeast infections. The rate of healthy bacteria in our bodies is decreased to levels where yeast can become overgrown. This occurs more often in women's bodies than in men's bodies. When either you or your boyfriend are taking an antibiotic, you may want to refrain from sexual activity and take a probiotic to promote the good bacteria in your body.

If neither of you were on an antibiotic—and you have no other reason why a yeast infection may be present—maybe your boyfriend sexually contracted the yeast infection from someone else and then transmitted it to you.

Q58

I seem to get UTIs a lot.
Can this be because of sex?

It could be; sexual activity is only one factor to consider when someone frequently gets UTIs (Urinary Tract Infections).

It is important to pee (yes, pee-pee, wiz, urinate, tinkle, whatever you prefer to call it) BEFORE and AFTER you have sexual intercourse to lower your risk of developing a UTI from any bacteria present during sexual intercourse.

Be sure to discuss with your doctor all possibilities of why the UTIs are occurring.

Q59

I was recently told I have HPV. Does this mean I will get genital warts at some point?

No. There are many strains of HPV and not all of them result in genital warts. Additionally, not all of the strains result in cervical cancer. Ask your doctor for more details about the strain you have and the corresponding symptoms.

In many cases, infections clear up within 2 years. In order for this happen, a stress-free, healthy lifestyle is suggested. That means getting 7-9 hours of a sleep each night, eating a balanced diet, getting at least 4 days of exercise in each week, and most importantly, avoiding stressful situations.

Taking good care of your health is beneficial in more ways than most people realize.

Q60

Does washing your penis after unprotected sex really work?

If you mean does it work to protect you against STIs/STDs or pregnancy, the answer is no.

Q61

I didn't understand the correlation between undiscovered STDs and cancer later on. Can you please repeat the information?

STDs/STIs that are undiagnosed and untreated can cause serious medical conditions including prostate cancer in men and cervical cancer in women. Many doctors and scientists feel that there is a link between STDs and prostate cancer, most likely due to inflammation resulting from an untreated STI.

HPV (Human Papillomavirus) is commonly associated with cervical cancer in women, but has also been linked to anal, oral, and penile cancers.

While you probably aren't interested in having kids right now, you may want them later and scarring from untreated STIs can result in infertility.

STIs can be transferred more easily between partners, because:

1. Symptoms are often short-term and can go unnoticed. If symptoms are noticed, many do not address the concern with a doctor.

2. Most sexually-active people do not get tested regularly.

3. Condom or other barrier protection is not always used.

4. There is no discussion about sexual history—
   the good, the bad, and the ugly experiences.
   We may not be proud of some of those
   experiences, but 80% of those infected will
   have no symptoms and 1 out of 5 teen girls
   contract an STI within one year of becoming
   sexually active!

Taking it a little further...

Early sexual activity and smoking can
double your risk of developing cancer
from a sexually transmitted infection/disease.

Human papillomavirus (HPV) can more
easily infect a young woman's cervix,
because the cells in the cervix
are still immature.

Smoking weakens the immune system.
Cigarette smoke contains chemicals
that can damage the body's cells
and cause them to become cancerous.

Because you keep asking...

Pregnancy

Yes, having a baby will change your life, but, don't think that having a child will provide you with unconditional love or the love of a boyfriend. This is a misconception of many young women. There has been some glamorization of teen pregnancy on TV shows and in the media. That's unfortunate and misleading, because pregnancy, having a baby, and raising a child is serious business.

Here's one of the most important factors that few people talk about: a woman's reproductive system is not fully developed until her early 20's, so why would anyone want to conceive a baby while there is still organ development to occur?

And yes, it is important to finish school. Yes, it costs a lot of money to have and raise a child. And no, it is not your parents' responsibility to raise or financially support your child.

You are responsible for your choices.
Do not downplay the serious consequences
attached to consensual sexual activity.

Instead of one careless night *or one selfish decision* that will instantaneously change your life forever, THINK, THINK, THINK, and then THINK AGAIN. Give yourself the time to discover yourself and the world around you, before you bring another life into this world.

Q62

Do you recommend that young women be on an oral birth control pill?

First and foremost, we recommend that women be educated about their reproductive health. The goal should be to prevent unintended pregnancies and for women to take an active role in their sexual health. We would not offer the blanket recommendation that most or all young women should be taking an oral contraceptive (OC) for numerous reasons:

* If you are not engaging in vaginal intercourse and don't plan to for some time, you don't need to be taking an OC.

* If you are forgetful, a medication that you need to take daily around the same time may not be a good idea. There are a lot of other contraceptive options that may better fit your style.

* We want to make sure to remind you that OC does not protect against STIs/STDs and should be used in conjunction with a barrier protection method if you want to practice safer sex.

* Oral contraceptives affect your hormone levels which affect many functions in your body. They can decrease sexual desire and affect who you find sexually desirable, by limiting your body's innate ability to receive those subtle messages about who you truly find appealing.

Q63

Can a girl get pregnant by "pre-cum?"

Yes. It's not like sperm have the ability to say, "Whoa, we can't go swimming yet, guys; he doesn't want us in there." Seminal fluid can contain sperm prior to ejaculation; this is why the "pull out" method is not a smart choice for avoiding pregnancy. Plus, without a condom, you have no barrier to protect against transmission of HIV, HPV, or any other STD/STI.

Note: Just for the sake of accuracy—there is a lubricating fluid that can exit the penis first. This fluid allows the semen to easily flow through the urethra. Since you won't be able to tell which fluid contains sperm and which does not, always play it safe.

Q64

I only had sex twice with this girl and she said she was on the pill... next thing I know she's telling me she's pregnant and wants to keep the baby. How did this happen?

This is one of the possible outcomes when you do not take personal responsibility for contraception.

Maybe the girl forgot to take her pill for a couple of days; maybe she was on another medication that interfered with the birth control; or get this... maybe she did not tell you the truth. Maybe she thought if she got pregnant, you would be her boyfriend. Lots of maybes... and yes, women have lied about birth control to trap men into a relationship. You would not be the first man to tell us this has happened.

No matter what a woman tells you—WEAR A CONDOM!! Or, how about this: don't have sex with anyone you would not want around for more than a couple nights.

Remember that oral contraceptives are not 100% effective when it comes to pregnancy (therefore, there was still a small chance she could become pregnant even if used correctly).

It only takes one time—perhaps even the first time. Now, because one sexual release was more important to you than protecting yourself, your future, and the future of an unplanned child, that woman and the baby will not only be a part of your world, but also your responsibility for the rest of your life.

It is now time for you to rise to the situation, be supportive to the mother, and be a great Dad. Be sure to tell your friends that the next time they desire a sexual release, they might want to find gratification by themselves or be sure to wear a condom.

Q65

I have heard that using EC or Plan B is like having an abortion. Is that true?

Excellent question, because the distinction is important. Using emergency contraception (EC) is very different from having an abortion.

The key with EC is that the woman is not already pregnant. EC works to boost the level of hormones in the body and prevent egg release (if one hasn't already been released) or by making the uterus inhospitable for egg implantation. If a woman happens to already be pregnant, EC will not harm the pregnancy.

If you do end up taking Plan B due to a broken condom, be prepared that the high level of estrogen in the medication can cause extreme breast swelling/tenderness and water-weight gain.

Please remember, Plan B is not intended as a regular or ongoing contraceptive option. It was designed to be used when another method works ineffectively.

Q66

What is the pregnancy rate on campus?

Good news: data from the Centers for Disease Control and Prevention's National Center for Health Statistics shows U.S. teen pregnancy rates have dropped since the 1990's.

Pregnancy rates for women in their early 20's declined to the lowest level in more than 3 decades.

More students receiving sexuality education in school and at home has played a big part in helping reduce the rate, along with increased access to birth control. We hope the information in this book continues to support the trend!

We thought it was important to include our thoughts on abortion, which has become more about politics rather than an opportunity to educate the public about avoiding unintended pregnancy.

We support women having a choice when it comes to childbearing. On occasion, abortion is part of the decision making process about whether to have any or more children.

We also support comprehensive sexuality education, which informs people of the numerous options available to help prevent unintended pregnancies. Our hope is that education will reduce the rate of unprotected sex, and as a result, decrease the rate of unintended pregnancies. Of course we realize that unprotected, consensual sex is not the only scenario that leads to unintended pregnancies; sexual assault is another reason we are pro-choice.

Our support of abortion as an available option for unwanted pregnancy by no means minimizes the seriousness of this medical procedure.

Though many women who have an abortion at a licensed facility do not experience any ill effects, as prevention educators, we want people to understand in advance the potential challenges associated with the procedure including: procedural discomfort/pain, emotional distress, and medical complications.

Abortion is a serious decision and should not be turned to casually as an alternative to an unwanted pregnancy. We hope most women won't have to make this decision. If you do, there are great resources to support you before, during, and after.

We invite you to join us in supporting comprehensive sexuality education and helping to reduce the need for abortion.

Because you keep asking...

Condoms

We love condoms! Male ones and female ones!

They are easy to find;

they do not require a prescription;

they are relatively inexpensive;

they are effective in helping to prevent
unintended pregnancy;

AND they decrease your risk of
contracting STIs/STDs.

Q67

Condoms keep breaking on me.
What do I do?

We are not having rough sex,
and we've tried different
brands and sizes.

Good job on doing your best to be safe. Not sure what you have already tried, so on the next page is a list of suggestions to help prevent breakage.

If you have already tried these suggestions, try using a female condom, but do not use a male and female condom at the same time.

To help prevent condom breakage:

» Check the expiration date; outdated
condoms break easier.

» Purchase a quality condom—and the size
that best fits you. Those with larger width
find that XL or Magnum™ condoms are
easier to put on.

» Put a small drop of water-based lubricant
on the top of the penis before rolling on
the condom. Too much lubricant may
cause the condom to slide off.

» Pinch any air out of the tip of the condom.

» Carefully roll on the condom without
putting nails through the condom. It's not
a good idea to put condoms on with your
teeth for they may make little shallow cuts
which later cause breakage.

» Put water-based lubricant on the outside
of the condom before penetration.

Q68

Do different types of condoms actually work differently in terms of pleasure?

They can work differently. There are many condom options, because people like options in regard to shape, size, color, texture, and sensation. Feel free to try a variety and see what works best for you and your partner.

Q69

My girlfriend thinks I need to use studded condoms. Does this reflect my performance?

No, it does not reflect your performance. Different condoms can make things fun and interesting. Most of us, tend to take things personally when it comes to sexual interactions with others. Relax, try something different, and see how you both like it. While this stuff can be serious, it is still supposed to be enjoyable!

Q70

How do you put on a condom? What happens if you put on a condom inside out?

The trick to knowing if you are putting a condom on "inside out" is that it does not go on as smoothly. See the answer to Q67 and review the "How to Use" Condom Video under Birth Control on the Planned Parenthood website.

If you have begun intercourse when you realize the mistake, throw the condom away and correctly put on a new one.

Do NOT turn the condom right side and continue having intercourse; there could be seminal fluid from inside the condom that now has an opportunity to enter the vagina.

Q71

Do condoms protect against everything?

Condoms can protect against *almost* everything when used properly.

Some quick, important notes:

1. Do not use condoms made from animal membranes, such as lambskin if you want to prevent HIV transmission. The HIV virus is small enough to transmit through the membrane.

   Be sure to use a latex or a poly-based condom to help prevent HIV transmission.

2. There are some STIs that are passed skin-to-skin. Therefore, even if you are using a condom, there is the chance that you could transmit or contract an STI/STD simply by rubbing the genital skin areas together.

3. While we always support people using condoms, male or female, it does not remove the need to have a conversation about health screenings and how to keep each other as healthy as possible.

Q72

How long should you wait before having sex without a condom if you have started taking birth control pills to avoid getting pregnant?

Medically, you need to wait one full cycle—take all 4 weeks of your pill pack before having sex without a condom to avoid unintended pregnancy.

Here is the caution:
Birth control pills do not protect you
from STIs/STDs.

We recommend that people use a barrier protection method (male condom, female condom, dental dam) until they are in a long-term, committed, monogamous relationship. If you are not yet in such a relationship, keep using a condom no matter how many months you have been taking the pill. It is just a good way to help stay healthy!

Taking it a little further...

To better understand the benefits,
and learn how to use female condoms
and dental dams, view the videos on
Planned Parenthood's website.

Q73

Do people have allergic reactions to condoms?

Yes. Many people are allergic to latex.

No worries, for there are polyisoprene and poly-urethane options available through most condom distributors.

Polyurethane transfers heat well and can be used with oil-based lubricants.

Polyisoprene is more natural feeling than poly-urethane, but cannot be used with oil-based lubricants.

For those of you using latex condoms: Latex can be weakened by certain lubricants so only water-based lubes should be used.

Other Good Stuff
(concerning the pelvic region)

Q74

How many times is too many times to masturbate in one day?

If you're asking this question, we're thinking you are concerned about the time you spend each day pleasuring yourself. Good for you for caring about your own well-being and asking a difficult question.

If you're asking us to give you a specific number, we'd say more than [an average of] three times in one day would cause us to question possible risk factors. *Where are you masturbating? In your room, car, public bathroom? Are you ditching classes to get off? Is this every day, and if so, how sore and red is the skin on your genitals? Are you concerned that you are beginning to exhibit addictive behaviors?*

Your questions about your sexual behavior are normal; 1 out of 4 students visit a counseling center for a question regarding sexuality.

We stand behind the theory that orgasm is beneficial to both women's and men's overall health. An orgasmic release via masturbation is exactly that—a release. Our oxytocin (naturally occurring drug that makes us feel happy) spikes and our sense of well-being is increased while tension is relieved, appetite is curbed, pain is decreased, sleep is improved, and the list goes on.

Q75

How do I convince a girl that my small penis doesn't affect the "motion of the ocean?"

B odies are different. Penis size and shape is different, vulva size and shape is different, the vaginal canal and uterus sit at different angles, and pelvic areas (hips, groin, butt) are different. How the two of you match up or fit together may affect what you consider the "motion of the ocean."

The truth is some people just physically fit better together. That said, you can still work on your technique by reading up on positions and how to be a better lover (hint: most women do not find the jack rabbit or freight train technique pleasant). Discuss with your girlfriend what she *does* like when you experiment.

Perhaps you will find that your concern about size is of little to no concern for your partner. As we have said other places in the book, we support the idea that you might date a number of people to find the "fit"—physically, mentally, and emotionally— that works well for you.

Q76

How do you tell if someone is interested in you or just wants to get laid?

A sk yourself questions such as:

1. How long has this person known me?

2. How much time have I spent with this person?

3. What authentic and kind gestures has this person expressed?

4. Does this person have a reputation for being "real" or full of it?

5. Am I interested enough to come right out and ask the person what they want from me?

6. What do I want from this person?

Q77

Why is it that men always feel the need to masturbate?

Part of that myth is driven by society. Not all men always feel the need to masturbate, but in their late teens, men's hormones can be at such a high level that the urge is more often on their minds. Getting sexually aroused or horny can happen more easily in youth than for men decades older.

Note: Women's hormones can also increase their desire for sexual release.

Q78

Is it true that if you watch a lot of porn, you won't be able to "get excited" when with a girl?

Well, if "watch a lot of porn" means you spend many hours each day or almost every day, then we could see a problem developing. We have met men of different ages who "watch a lot of porn" and seem to have lost touch with reality when it comes to women and sexual behavior.

In sexually explicit films, sexual acts are not a depiction of reality. What happens before the director yells "Action!" is not seen on camera. There is extensive time spent on both the male and female to prep them for sexual activity.

And, a lot of the *oohs* and *aahs* expressed by the actors are just that—acting. Touching a women's elbow is not going to cause her to scream in ecstasy, but we have seen this take place in XXX films.

Real human contact, real life loving situations should be the goal. Yes, we all need a fantasy here or there to provoke excitation, but if you're living in a fantasy world, you're going to be continually disappointed when real life doesn't measure up.

Q79

Can all girls ejaculate?

When a woman's urethral sponge (which rests above the vaginal canal) is massaged, she can ejaculate fluid. In order for this to take place, the glands enmeshed within the urethral tissue must be stimulated correctly and the women must be able to "let go" and allow the fluid to be released. (No, the clear, watery fluid is not urine.)

Women are all different. Some will welcome the idea and others will have no interest. There are many women who have never experienced it nor believe they are not capable of ejaculation.

Q80

How do you make a guy last longer during sex?

Quick ejaculation could be caused by premature ejaculation issues (when a male's sexual climax—orgasm—occurs in less than 2 minutes or when it occurs before desired).

Premature ejaculation is common among sexually inexperienced males simply due to lack of knowledge of how their body works. It can also be caused by certain drugs (even over-the-counter ones), stress, anxiety, or psychological issues.

Determining what is influencing premature ejaculation is key to helping the guy last longer. In some cases, a product rubbed or sprayed on the penis can be effective. There is also a squeeze technique which you can learn to assist your guy. Above all, be patient. With both of you addressing the situation, it should improve.

Taking it a little further...

For information on the squeeze technique:
GoAskAlice.columbia.edu

Q81

Does taking steroids or medications affect the penis?

Yes and yes. Steroids and medications can cause all sorts of sexual problems or dysfunction.

Steroids are artificial testosterone, so when you take steroids your body reduces the natural production of testosterone. Some steroids can cause Erectile Dysfunction (no hard-on or a hard-to-maintain hard-on) or the inability to have an orgasm.

Note: Be cautious of what you read in some body-building forums. Also, be careful with what you are putting into your body in your attempt to increase muscle size and/or fitness level.

Medications, along with alcohol, marijuana, and pain killers can also affect your sexual health in the following ways:

» decreased desire   » hormone imbalances

» erection issues   » depression

» no orgasm   » fatigue

Aren't these consequences enough to avoid careless usage of these substances?

Q82

Does ejaculation decrease testosterone?
Does it hurt post workout muscle recovery?

L et's tackle these questions separately.

Testosterone levels may rise slightly during sexual activity (including masturbation), but levels return to normal thereafter.

After a workout, you want your muscles to relax so they can heal and become stronger. Sexual activity requires some work; therefore, fooling around and ejaculation wouldn't allow the body to rest. If you're with your significant other, your performance most likely won't be your best!

Q83

Does it hurt the most when a girl has sex for the first time?

Sex should never ever, ever, ever hurt—during the first time or the 5th time or the 50th time. If there is pain or discomfort, your body is telling you that something is "wrong" or "off."

Reasons for discomfort or pain:

- Anxiety is not allowing the body to relax.

- Lack of foreplay is not allowing the cervix/uterus to lift and the vaginal canal to become lubricated.

- There is lack of lubrication due to delayed physiological response related to alcohol, drugs, marijuana, medication, or illness.

- Your partner is rough or inconsiderate.

- You have not acquired enough knowledge, experience, or understanding about your body and sexuality.

- There may be a physical abnormality that needs to be checked out by a gynecologist.

- There is a lack of "fit" between you and your partner's body; the 2 of you simply do not fit well together.

Q84

Please explain to the guys that girls have 3 holes not 2!

Yep. Guys, the 3 "holes" are:

> The Urethra
>> The Vagina
>>> The Anus

Guys, you urinate and ejaculate semen out of your urethra, but a women's urethra is only used for urination.

Q85

Is it a bad idea to have sex with someone in your res hall?

The answer depends on how you set it up and who you choose as your sex partner.

If you choose someone who is looking for a relationship and you lead them to believe you are too (when you're not), then don't be surprised when the awkwardness or revenge takes place.

If you have a transparent discussion about your intentions, and find your neighbor is in agreement, then you have reduced the risk of fallout.

Remember, getting horizontal and naked with someone can change the dynamics of a relationship quite quickly, even if you have the best of intentions.

Q86

What is a realistic number of people on college campuses who are sexually active?

It's about half and half. About half of your fellow students are NOT engaging in sexual activity. Some are waiting for marriage, some are waiting for a relationship *with* strings, some want to avoid accidental pregnancy, and others are more concerned with their school work and want to avoid relationship drama.

With media influences and peers boasting about getting laid, it can be difficult to talk about your choice to not be sexually active.

There is no such thing as "have to"—you don't have to be sexually active in college. Don't allow anyone to make you feel as though you are missing something; there is no expiration on sexual desire.

The double standard still exists. Guys are often congratulated for having sex with multiple girls, while females are usually regarded as "sluts" if they have had sexual activity outside of a committed relationship or marriage. The word "slut" means "promiscuous" which means "one's sexual activity is not restricted to one partner." Hmmm... doesn't "slut" define the guys having sex with multiple women?

Q87
What do you do if your partner is too big?

Mainly, we want you to avoid painful experiences and respect your own needs. Did you know that a woman with a tilted forward uterus can comfortably handle a larger penis or toy than a woman with a tilted backward uterus?

**Women are different sizes
just as men are different sizes.**

Always allow your body time to warm up. When you allow your body the time to prepare, the cervix draws up higher in the vaginal canal in preparation for intercourse; this is helpful if length is the issue. If width is the issue, always use lube with protection, but there might be the realization not everyone fits well together.

Another important factor to remember is that if you tear the vaginal mucosa, you increase the chances of an STI/STD being transmitted. If penetration hurts, stop intercourse immediately. You may want to speak with a doctor to ensure there is no inflamation causing a problem.

Q88

What should I do if there is a lot of pubic hair?

A variation in the amount of pubic hair on men and women is totally normal. Some people like to leave it natural and some remove it all. Others prefer a well-trimmed look that can take many shapes—landing strip, heart, tree, teardrop, etc.

If you prefer less hair, offer to do some trimming for your partner. There are small electric razors that have tips to prevent cutting sensitive skin.

If your partner insists on keeping it wild... we understand certain activities such as oral sex may be less appetizing—getting hair in your teeth isn't much fun. Try smoothing the hair out of the way with your hand and hold your hand in that place while [hopefully] enjoying the experience.

Q89

Do you think it's wrong to lead a girl on when you don't want her to be your girlfriend, but want the constant hook-up?

If you are pretending you want her to be your girlfriend, then the answer is yes. You already knew that. *Do you like it when people are dishonest with you?*

Tell her you are only interested in the available hookup. Then, it's her choice whether she wants to take part. This is one of the situations where we set ourselves up for failure because someone always gets hurt or has different expectations.

Intimacy causes certain biological sequences to occur that make "casual sex" anything but casual. You can pretend it's just a hookup, but relationships and sexual activity have far more reaching effects. You're better off with your available hand in your room alone.

Q90
Is having sex while the girl is menstruating unhealthy?

There is no medical reason for vaginal intercourse during menstruation to be unhealthy; menstrual flow is just a bodily fluid. Points of consideration would be if she feels comfortable having sex at this time and be aware there can be increased vaginal discharge.

Practicing safer sex is especially important when a girl is experiencing a heavy period flow. Vaginal pH is less acidic during this time, increasing the chances of a yeast or bacterial infection such as bacterial vaginosis.

Note: During mentruation, a woman's risk of contracting an STI/STD is higher than normal—the cervix opens to allow blood to pass through, creating an opportunity for bacteria to reach further into the vaginal canal. And, diseases such as HIV and hepatitis are more likely to be passed on to a partner.

Menstruating is not a free pass to have unprotected sex; there is still a chance you could become pregnant depending on the day of her cycle and how long her cycle lasts.

Q91

I don't know what my vagina looks like. Should I know?

A bsolutely! We encourage everyone to be familiar with his or her own body; you should know more about it than anyone else. Get a better understanding of your vulva by checking it out while you are in the shower or bath. You could also use a hand mirror and spend a little time identifying your outer and inner labia, clitoris, clitoral hood, and vaginal opening.

Know that outer and inner labia come in all sorts of shapes and sizes. The names can be confusing, but most women will have inner lips (labia minora) that extend beyond the labia majora (outer lips). The labia are usually asymmetrical just as a man's testicles do not hang even.

Don't get caught up in porn star labia where the women have often had labiaplasty to surgically alter the size of their lips. The procedure can result in scar tissue and decreased sensitivity in an area that naturally responds to touch.

One last thought... women's vulvas are beautiful. They represent pleasure, love, and birth of life!

A common misconception is that females have a "vagina" as males have a penis. Women do have a vagina; it is part of their vulva. Vulva is the correct term.

Q92

Is there such a thing as having too much sex?

There are responsibilities in life: work, school, family, friends, living environment, etc. If you are enjoying a sexually active lifestyle but can still complete other responsibilities *on time and successfully*, then it sounds like you have achieved a healthy balance.

Our question to you is, "Is this with multiple partners?" Frequency is one thing, but having multiple partners and increasing your risk for becoming infected with HPV, STIs/STDs, or AIDS is another.

Be sure to listen to your body; if you (or your partner) are sore or feel a UTI (urinary tract infection) coming on, then be sure to allow the body time to rest and heal. Inflamed, irritated skin may increase your chance of infection.

Taking it a little further...

6 oral sex partners in your lifetime
makes YOU
3 times as likely to get oral cancer

We would like to take a moment to address the term Intersex. Intersex is a term that describes a variety of conditions when a person is born with chromosomes that vary from the expected XX-female or XY-male chromosomes. When a person is born with such a variation, the sexual and/or reproductive anatomy does not seem to fit the typical definitions of male or female.

There is quite a variety of chromosomal difference and while some of the results of that difference can be seen at birth, there are many occasions where it may not be known until the time puberty usually begins and can possibly go undetected over an entire lifetime.

1 in every 1500-2000 babies
is born intersexual.

Taking it a little further...

For detailed information, visit:
The Intersex Society of North America

www.isna.org

---

*Here is some biology trivia for you:
Did you know that the default gender of a fetus is female? All babies start out as female!

When there is a Y chromosome, the brain uses the female hormone estradiol to "masculinize" the brain, which then releases male hormones to develop male organs. For example, the tissue that would become an ovary in a female becomes a testicle and descends. Think about this: What happens when the brain doesn't complete the "masculinization" process?

We all have an X chromosome: two X's make a female; one X and one Y makes a man. Ha! Any man is half a woman!

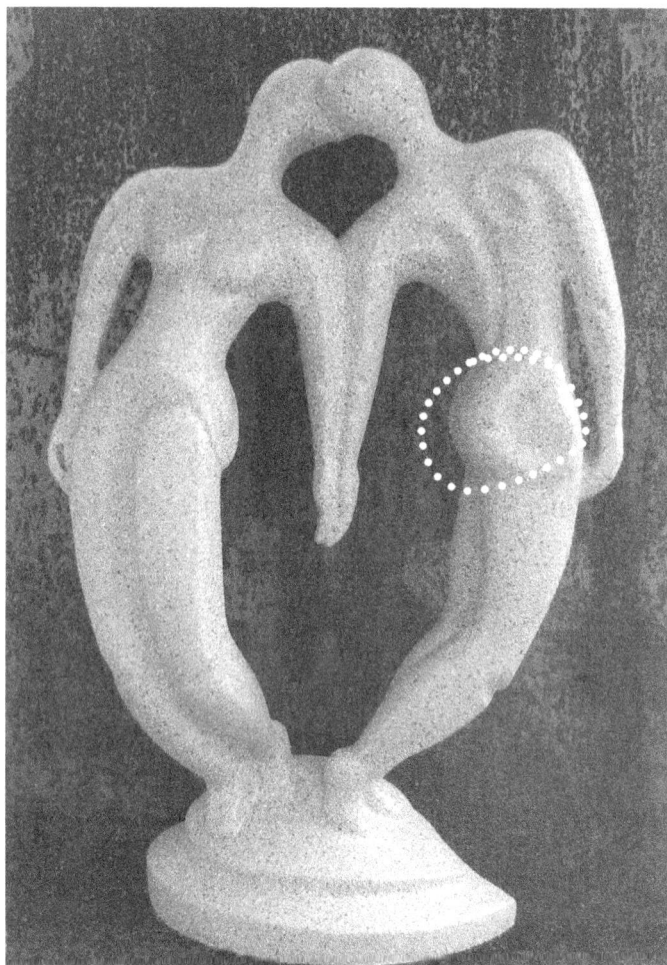

BUTT
Questions dealing with
our anal opening,
anus, rectum...

Anal sex is another form of sex. Some people feel anal sex is an alternative to penile/vaginal intercourse if they want to remain a virgin. Others challenge the concept that you can have anal sex and still call yourself a virgin. It depends on how you define virginity. You may believe any form of sex (anal, vaginal, oral) qualifies as losing one's virginity. Remember, sexuality is as varied and complicated as the human mind.

It is estimated less than 10% of heterosexual couples regularly engage in anal sex. We felt it was important to include these questions to ensure students have the correct information, before making a decision that affects their sexual health.

Q93

Why do men feel pleasure through anal sex? Do women like it?

The capacity to enjoy anal sex is available to everyone. We all have sensory receptors in our anus; and some people like the way it feels when that area is stimulated during sexual activity. While some people find it a turn on, others find it a turn off.

Two reasons men may particularly enjoy anal sex include:

1. If they are penetrating, the sphincters of the anus may be tighter than that of a mouth or a vagina and the increased pressure felt during penetration is pleasurable.

2. If they are being penetrated, the easiest way to provide pressure to the prostate gland is through the rectum. Pressure to the prostate gland is often noted as being very pleasurable and is regularly said to be the male equivalent of the female g-spot.

Q94

Should you use a condom during anal sex?

Always! It is easier to break blood capillaries in the anus and therefore increases the probability of transmitting an infection.

You can use a male or female condom for anal sex. Female condoms, which are an option for vaginal intercourse, were orginally invented for anal sex.

Q95

How can you make anal sex more comfortable and enjoyable?

By taking it extremely slow and making sure both partners are comfortable with what is happening.

There are products on the market that help to numb the skin surrounding the anus with the intention of making penetration smoother/possible, but we do not believe you should have to desensitize yourself for a sexual act. There is also "foreplay" needed to prepare the anus for penetration.

If you decide you want to try to work towards feeling more comfortable, then start small. Try playing with a finger or small toy before moving onto a large toy or penile penetration.

If it feels uncomfortable at any time, find another option.

Most people do not understand the proper foreplay and preparation necessary before engaging in anal sex. Fecal matter is toxic, yes TOXIC, so you may decide to more thoroughly cleanse the rectum with an enema prior to anal play.

If you are suffering from hemorrhoids, fissures or tears, do not engage in anal sex until you have consulted with a physician. If anal sex interests you, do your homework to avoid literally having or being a pain in the butt.

Taking it a little further...

It is best to allow a few hours to pass after an enema before anal sex.

Even if using soap and water to clean the anus, be careful for soap can be harsh and cause small tears that increase the risk of contracting an STI/STD.

NEVER insert a penis or sex toy into the mouth or vagina after it's been inserted in the rectum. Be sure to use a new condom and clean sex toys in between.

Q96

Can you get a girl pregnant through anal sex?

It's a long shot, but not totally impossible. There is no internal function connecting the rectum to the vagina, fallopian tubes, or uterus; therefore, if you were to ejaculate into a woman's anal canal, the sperm could not travel internally for conception to take place.

However, what could happen is that ejaculate could come out of her anus and seep into her vaginal canal and potentially result in pregnancy. While this is unlikely to happen, it is not impossible due to the closeness of the anus and the vaginal canal.

An important note: With unprotected anal sex, there is a high risk of contracting/transferring a sexually transmitted infection, because the bacteria in the anus can enter the urethral opening. There is also an increased rate of bladder infections in women. It is good to get in the habit of cleaning the urethra and the vulva after sexual activity.

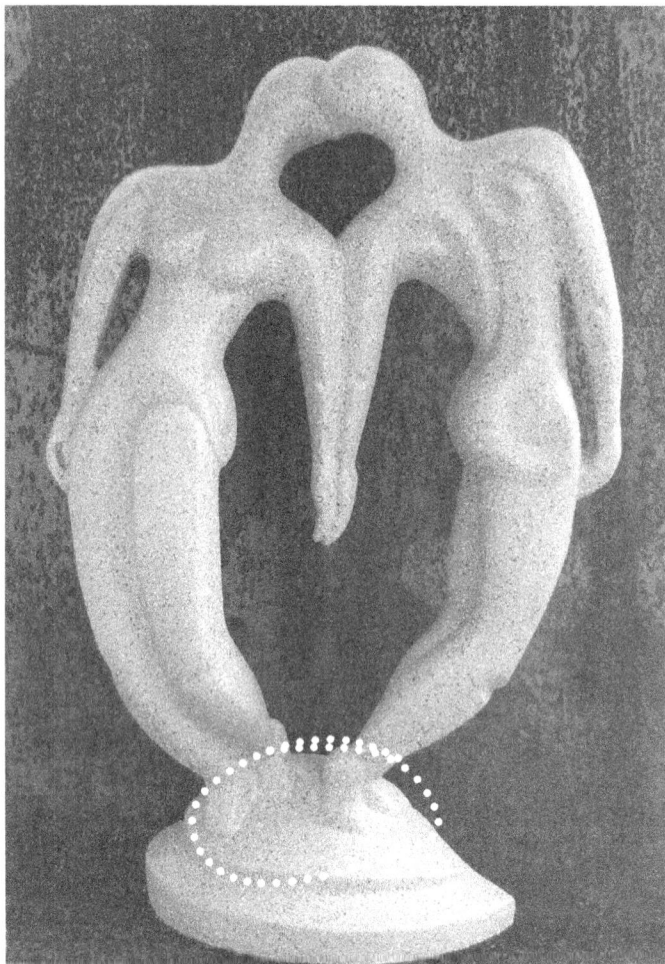

TOES
Questions dealing with
self-worth & self respect

No, this section is not about foot fetishes; it is about standing up for yourself, standing up for others, and standing on your own two feet. It's about having the courage to be the one to say or do something when no one else will.

Self-worth and self-respect play a part in every aspect of your life. Think about those words...

Self-worth
Self-respect

What do you think you are "worth?"
What do you deserve in life?

Only YOU can answer those questions for yourself, but we'll tell you this:

* Everyone has worth.

* Have faith in yourself.

* You deserve whatever you give to others.

* And, at some point, you will need to find
  30 seconds of courage when no one else can.

Q97

Why do boyfriends promise to treat you better when you get back together, and do for a short period of time, then change back to treating you badly?

This answer is simple: because he can. For some reason, you call someone "boyfriend" who treats you poorly. You throw a hissy fit, break up with him and then you love that he comes crawling back, promising to treat you better. Of course, he goes right back to the way he has *always* treated you. It is all he is capable of and on some level you know you deserve better.

Good for you for wanting to be treated with kindness; now do something serious about the situation. Repeat after us:

> "(His Name), this isn't working out
> for me. You and I are not compatible.
> I wish you luck in finding someone who
> is a better match."

Q98

How should someone handle a significant other whose actions are often hurtful, but he (or she) always comes around to apologize profusely for his (or her) actions?

Is it okay to always forgive him (or her)?

The worrisome part of your question is "often hurtful." Why are you choosing to be with someone who does not care about your well-being and happiness? We all make mistakes and shoot off our mouth at one time or another; therefore, it is important to apologize and seek forgiveness. If however, someone continually chooses to do the same hurtful thing over and over and over again, the apologies seem empty and not very authentic.

Forgive and move on to someone who genuinely cares about you. Stop allowing "friends" to stomp all over your feelings; you deserve better. Find friends who treat you as you treat them.

Q99

Why do guys play games?
Why don't they just say
"I like you" or "I don't like you?"

Wouldn't that be great if people could just be honest and transparent about how they feel? Unfortunately, emotions sometimes make us feel uncomfortable and inhibit us from verbally expressing our true feelings. It's not like in the movies where the guy shows up at the girl's office and proclaims in front of everybody how much he is in love with her.

The games you are referring to are about power and control and not wanting to appear desperate. At some point, you have to decide how much of the game you are willing to play:

- *Are you ok with him showing you affection one day and blowing you off the next?*

- *Are you satisfied with booty calls only?*

- *Are you ok that he wants to see other girls?*

- *Are you willing to put up with him flaking on you when he promised to show up?*

Dating and relationships have a learning curve. Love & Learn. If someone is playing too many games with your head, you may want to find someone who plays *with you* instead of against you.

Q100

How do I help my friend who is in an abusive relationship? She downplays the negative aspects when things aren't that bad.

It is typical for a person in an abusive relationship to forget about the abuse when everything is going well. Offer continual support to your friend, so she knows you will be there for her when things get bad again (and they will).

Suggest that meeting with a therapist/counselor may help strengthen their relationship. Most abused women do not have the strength or desire to give up on the relationship right away.

Look for physical signs such as bruising. You can anonymously report the abusive boyfriend if she refuses to get help. It is important to alert administrators in order to protect you, your friend, and all students on campus. Though you may be saving her life, she may see you as the enemy because "you just don't understand their kind of love."

There is no abusive behavior in a healthy, loving relationship. Thank you for being a good friend and caring about her well-being and safety.

Q101

I have a friend who is dating a man who doesn't respect or pay attention to her. We have had conversations about it, but she still stays with him.

How can I help her realize that she doesn't have to "settle" for him?

Relationships are about choices. We're glad to see you have a strong sense of self-worth; unfortunately, your friend's self-worth is nowhere to be found. She most likely has thoughts similar to, "no one else will love me if I lose this guy." It will be hard for you to watch her stay in this relationship, but it is her choice whether or not she chooses a fabulous guy or someone who uses her.

Many young women today fail to recognize that when they do not respect themselves, they only attract the type of guy who does not care whether or not his girlfriend's heart is happy. It's all about him and his needs. Not all men are taught to respect women; and society's tolerance of disrespectful behavior is not helping the situation.

You may decide to spend less time with this friend. (That's OK.) Choosing to surround yourself with friends who support your emotional well-being and their own well-being is always a good idea.

You have already approached her about your concerns; maybe the words of wisdom would have a greater impact coming from someone else. The book *I AM before "I DO"* may be the perfect gift for your friend.

What is Respect in a Relationship?

* Do you value each other's feelings, thoughts, and ideas?

* Do you have admiration for each other and avoid comments that suggest he or she is: dumb, ugly, over/underweight, or unworthy of love?

* Do you exhibit manners towards one another?

* Do you both show consideration for each other's gender, race, culture, and family?

Final thoughts...

A s you've read, sexuality is complex. We did our best to answer your questions succinctly and hope you never stop asking questions about what you don't know.

Check out the wellness or health center on campus or visit SmartSexRocks.com for resources.

Love Well, Live Well,
Ranee & Kim

Healthy Attitude towards Sexuality = Healthy You

Love & Light to the following individuals who have in some way helped to make this book reach the millions of students who we serve:

Vinnie & Jolene Amoroso
Debbie Bazarsky
Rick Belling
Eric Benedetti
Connie Bowes
Stephanie Buehler
John & Dawn Chestnut
Cayla Conover
Nicole Counts
Melanie Davis
Andy Doan
Cameron Dumas
Susanne Fest
Debbie & Larry Gustafson
HEART Peer Educators
Angel Lozzi
Chris & Natalie Lozzi

Bekah Martinez
Mark Mikelat
Hannah Mitchell
Savanah Moore-Kondo
Steve Morita
Lawrence Ogunka
Enoh Okodiko
Stacy Rini
Joh Robbins
Jillian Shih
Karen Snyder
Terese Sergi & Family
Joe & Grace Spina
Jason Steich
Lisa Taxin
Brandon Thompson
Stephanie Youssef

*Special thanks to Lisa Kazanjian, our goddess of editing, for ensuring we had our commas and semi-colons appropriately placed!

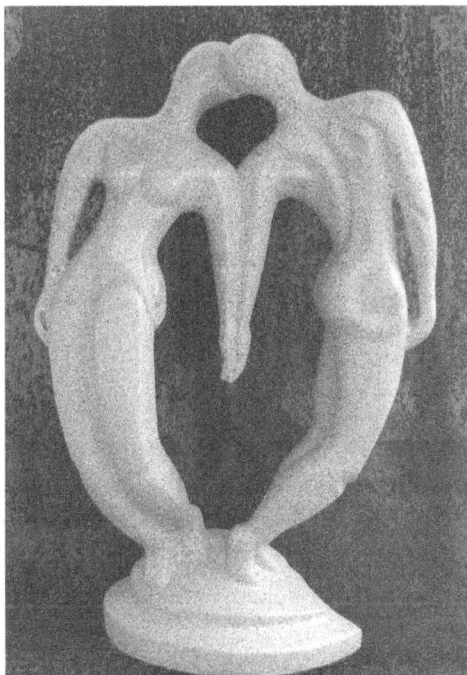

Heart Couple Statue
by Mike Jensen
Zhki's Gallery
www.zhkis.com

About the Authors

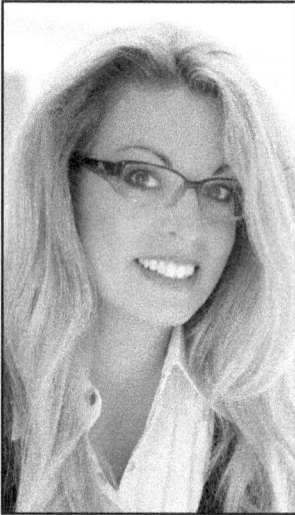

Ranee Alison Spina is a speaker and author of the two-time Award-Winning *I AM before "I DO" - Unsolicited Advice on LOVE*.

She strives to be a catalyst for her audiences with humorous, uncompromising honesty about sexuality and relationship issues.

Ranee's passionate, interactive campus lecture *Understanding SEX & LOVE* is life-changing and truly entertaining. At heart, when she steps on stage, Ranee is still that rockstar who performed on the Sunset Strip in Los Angeles years ago.

She now resides by the beach in Orange County, California.

Follow Ranee for Wellness and Sexual Health Tips.
Twitter: @rockin_sex_ed
Instagram: rockinsexed
Facebook: Ranee Alison Spina

About the Authors

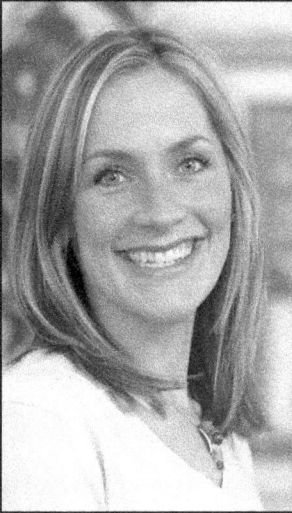

Dr. Kimberly Chestnut is presently a Human Sexuality and Health Education Professor at a university in Philadelphia, where she also is the Director of Student Wellness.

Due to the success of her campus and community wellness programs, she is often asked to present at industry trainings and conferences.

Kimberly warmly welcomes students into her office who have endless questions about sexual health, and her ultimate goal is to share the beautiful complexity of sexuality around the world.

Kimberly currently resides in Pennsylvania and loves participating in triathlons, supporting wildlife preservation, and sharing time with her husband, Jason, and their yellow lab, Jackson.

www.ingramcontent.com/pod-product-compliance
Lightning Source LLC
Chambersburg PA
CBHW021159010426
R18062100001B/R180621PG41931CBX00035B/63